Beware of Falling Coconuts

Beware of Falling Coconuts

GILLIAN MCNEILL

Published in 2019 by Gillian McNeill

With the help of Lumphanan Press
9 Anderson Terrace, Tarland
Aberdeenshire, AB34 4YH
www.lumphananpress.co.uk

Printed and bound by Imprint Digital,
Upton Pyne, Devon.

ISBN: 978-1-5272-4520-4

Dedicated to Louie, Maureen, Moyra & Janet

Contents

Introduction

A NUMBER OF YEARS AGO I visited the beautiful Caribbean island of Jamaica. I was staying in Montego Bay and one day, on my way to the beach, I saw a hand painted sign which said, 'Beware of Falling Coconuts'. It stopped me in my tracks. I had never thought about a coconut being dangerous before, but apparently coconuts kill more people than sharks... fifteen times more people. A silent predator, hanging in wait. Without warning it can attack, dropping from a great height at a ferocious speed. At that moment a voice in my head told me, 'This is the title of a book you are going to write'. It took me by surprise because I had no burning desire to write a book. Writers wrote books and I was not a writer. I certainly didn't think that I would one day be writing about another silent and much feared predator: cancer.

Nowadays, most people you meet are affected, either directly or indirectly, by cancer. The thing is, when you've come through it and survived, or know someone who has, it makes you want to give something back. Most of us have participated in some way, or at least thought about it, to raise money for cancer charities or cancer research. There's no end to the weird and wacky ideas. Those who go sober for October, then cannae remember November. Those who buy cakes, bake cakes, and eat cakes. Those who hold coffee mornings and participate in a slice of life, and those who brave the shave, from top to bottom. (On the subject of bottoms, I include the full monty in that!) They dare to bare, whilst some choose to donate their hair. Then there are the 5k, 10k, midnight walkers and kilt walkers... those cycling or racing for life, the bloggers and the joggers wearing yellow or pink t-shirts, tutus, wristbands, bows, deely-boppers, and daffodils. No matter what it is, we all have one thing in common and that is the desire to help other people.

During my illness I was fortunate to meet some inspiring people... some who are sadly no longer with us. Despite the black cloud of cancer hanging over them they showed me that sometimes there was laughter to be found even in the most bizarre situations.

As well as family members, I lost a friend and colleague, Lesley Fitz-Simons to the disease. I met Lesley when we were both young actresses working at Scottish Television filming Take the High Road. We shared a dressing room, we socialised together and even went on holiday together. During that time we shared a lot of champagne and a lot of laughter. That's what I remember about Lesley, her infectious laughter. Over the years, work and family life took us in different directions and we lost touch. However, we met by chance a few months before she died and she told me about her cancer. It was actually a very positive conversation. She spoke about the happiness her daughter and partner gave her and she was keen to share her stories and hear mine. Although she was clearly in pain, she still managed to find plenty to laugh about.

I remember how encouraged I was and how positive I felt after listening to a woman who claimed comedy cured her cancer. However far-fetched that sounds, I certainly know that humour helped me through mine. I hope that, as you read this, you will find something in it to make you smile, because this is my way of giving something back. After all, they do say laughter is the best medicine!

Howkin Tatties

As a child I was extremely well endowed. I had been blessed with two huge, red swellings that filled the back of my throat. They were regularly infected and looked like the surface of the moon. Deep craters, filled up with all sorts of nasties, causing me no end of problems, and I've still got them.

My daughter Molly inherited the same gargantuan obstacles at the back of her throat; they flared up, grew yellow spots and oozed hard globules of pus with increasing frequency. Yet still they were not keen to remove them. Thank God she didn't get my bunions!

June 2015 was an exceptionally busy month for us. Molly was to start primary seven after the summer holidays at a new school and she was nervously anticipating the approaching taster day, combined with having to say goodbye to old friends and worrying about making new ones. But that wasn't all that was occupying her thoughts. There were always the tonsils, the bane of our lives. Like most parents I will never forget the week she eventually got them removed. It's typical but whenever there is a drama in our house it always seems to happen when Alan is working away, this time on a remote Scottish island with no wi-fi or phone reception.

Three days is a long time to stay in hospital after a tonsillectomy, but the surgeon had remarked on how difficult they had been to remove due to their size, and he felt it wise to keep her under observation in case of a bleed.

'Reminded me of the backbreaking labour of howkin tatties as a bairn,' he remarked. I tried not to form that picture in my mind. Thank God I didn't have to watch!

Quite frankly, it was a bit tedious sitting and staring at a blank wall while Molly slept. Not having planned for an extended stay, the book I had brought was long finished and, whilst she had the advantage of being the only patient in an empty ward in a brand-new hospital, it meant that some facilities were not yet available. I stared at the huge bracket that had just been mounted on the wall opposite, imagining the flat screen TV that would shortly be attached to it. Daytime TV had never seemed more appealing. Not even a free newspaper or an out-of-date magazine had made it into the ward. The shops and cafes were in the process of being stocked so the catering facilities consisted of a vending machine.

However, the advantage of being the only patient in the ward was that the medical care was fantastic, and that's all that really mattered. Looking back, I should have practiced mindfulness and been grateful for the lull before the storm.

The following morning I was supposed to have a well woman appointment and mammogram at the old Western Infirmary on the other side of the city. I debated cancelling it as I didn't want to leave Molly alone in the hospital, but the nurses persuaded me to go. I had been to my GP with a lump in my right breast, which had since grown to the size of a small plum. I wasn't unduly alarmed as I have gristly boobs so finding pea-sized lumps was a regular occurrence. This, however, was bigger than usual and it had been there for a few months, so it was wise to get it checked. Fortunately that morning one of the doctors popped her head in early, before starting her rounds, to see how Molly was doing.

Happy with the healing she discharged Molly and told me I had to take her straight home for bedrest.

'Oh God,' I thought. 'What do I do?'

Molly wanted to be with me and yet I had waited ages for the appointment, I couldn't cancel it. I had no choice but to take her with me. So the poor wee soul was bundled into the car and driven over to a draughty old hospital where just a few skeleton clinics were running... and I don't mean for bones.

I was scared she would catch an infection. She was still very sore and weak and needed to be at home tucked up in her warm bed. I may sound a bit paranoid but by this time I was living on my nerves. The only people I could contact to collect Molly were relatives who lived in East Kilbride, about forty minutes' drive away. Fortunately her Auntie Linda and Uncle Paul, who Molly adored and who I knew would take good care of her, dropped everything and jumped in the car straight away. We arranged that they would collect Molly from the reception of the Western Infirmary and take her home.

I had been warned that I could be waiting for a long time as the clinic was a one stop shop for everything: mammograms, X-rays, biopsies... you name it, they did it.

I will never forget her little face when I was called through and I had to leave her sitting all alone. I begged the non-plussed receptionist to look after her. Huddled in a coat with a small overnight bag at her feet and the whitest, palest, most frightened expression on her face, I told her not to move till Auntie Linda arrived. As I walked away down the long empty corridor I could never have imagined that, just a few short hours later, she wouldn't be the only one sitting alone in a waiting room with a ghostly white pallor.

A Diamond Diagnosis

THERE'S NO DOUBT ABOUT IT, when you receive a cancer diagnosis it's numbing. Which, looking back, was actually a blessing. It allowed time for my brain to process the devastating blow.

My diagnosis was confirmed by a rather apologetic-looking doctor, who was reading my ultrasound notes and images and glancing at x-rays before the door swung open and the big guns rolled in. You know they're a high heid yin when they're a Miss or a Mister, not just a Doctor. Mine was a Miss and she had an air of serious doom about her as she delivered the verdict. Obviously not known for her gentle bedside manner, all that was missing was a black cap as she pronounced judgement and passed sentence upon me.

'Give me a year of your life, and I will give you your life.'

I can't really remember the conversation that followed. I felt like a child sitting in the headmaster's office. This was serious, this was really happening to me. So, why was I not reacting? What was I doing? Nothing to say? No questions?

I couldn't take my eyes off the giant diamonds on her left-hand ring finger. Not just one or two, but lots of them, twinkling and flashing as she drew circles on the sketch of a human breast. I was mesmerised by dazzling crosses and shimmering arrows pointing to the under arm, then RHS (right hand side) was scribbled in a blaze of glorious, sparkling technicolour. All the time she was talking about courses of treatment and waiting for results or something, but the diamonds were moving so quickly and I kept losing count and having to start again. How many carats were on that finger? Were they all hers? Was she a married 'Miss' or were they her mother's, a family heirloom perhaps? She must have come from a wealthy family. What did her husband do for a living? Why presume a husband? Should I have complimented her on the diamonds? Asked to try them on?

I didn't have a clue what she said, what was happening, or indeed the order of events in those first few days. I was forty-nine years old and I had been excited about turning a fabulous fifty in September. All of a sudden everything changed as I was faced with my own mortality check. I was a mum. I was a wife. It couldn't be happening to us. The surrealness of the situation took over and like a prisoner I was processed into their system, all choice and decision-making taken from me as I was passed from room to room and tested and biopsied and x-rayed and mammogramed. I was like a battery hen. All that was missing was a barcode and some packaging and I would have been ready for the nearest poultry section of the supermarket. Me just lying there with the other plump white chicken breasts, waiting to be prodded and squeezed and analysed. Hoping I wasn't past my sell by date... although I was definitely *best before* all this.

Panini Machine

As I lay in the dimly lit room with just a long sheet of paper tissue for warmth and dignity, I realised I had no idea how a biopsy would feel. A word of warning girls... when the lovely doctor sticks a needle in your boob and asks you to tell her if the anaesthetic is starting to work, say *NO*. Shout for more anaesthetic. In my naivety I said my boob was numb, hoping to speed things along. I certainly did not want a dead arm either, because I had to drive home. I had to go to the supermarket, make dinner, get home to Molly. Big mistake!

As she started to perform the biopsy the pain was acute. I had always prided myself on my high pain threshold. I gave birth with gas and air for God's sake, so why was a needle in the boob so bloody painful? Was I becoming a wimp? How many holes was she making with that needle? I was being turned into a human watering can. I started to invent little scenarios to distract myself from the pain. If I took a drink of water would it come pouring out the holes in my chest? I was sure I had seen something like that on Laurel and Hardy as a child. Funny what comes into your head at times of stress.

With my biopsy complete it was off for a mammogram. I tell you, if I wasn't needing a mastectomy at that particular moment, I would bloody well need one by the time they were finished. A purple and red mass was spreading over my breast area and the ultrasoundogropher person (a technical term) was quite alarmed.

'Oh dear, that's quite a mess we have made of you. Sorry... it's just bruising. Are you sore? You should have said and had more anaesthetic. You will know the next time.'

Next time? I hadn't been planning a next time. Ignorance is bliss as they say because yes, there was indeed a next time. Further biopsies were taken from surrounding tissue and lymph nodes. I was also to have a clip inserted, apparently to measure any growth of the tumour, or plum as I preferred to call it. What was wrong with the bloody tape measure the other doctor used? Let's face it, the plum was big enough... six centimetres at the last recording. It's not like they wouldn't be able to find it. Perhaps they should have microchipped me at the same time in case I ever got lost in the system. Visions of a banana clip type of contraption filled my mind. How the hell were they going to get something that size inside my boob? I decided not to ask. I just hoped that whoever was doing it was a fully paid up member of the magic circle. As far as I was concerned, it was going to take a bloody magician to perform that trick.

I closed my eyes and prayed that the anaesthetic was super-charged. Then, with a wee wave of her magic wand and a puff of smoke, my clip was in place. I didn't feel a thing. And the only thing that could possibly follow that performance? Yip! You guessed! I was off for another mammogram.

Now ladies, you know how we don't tell the younger gener-ation horror stories about childbirth, because we don't want to freak them out? Well, mammograms should come with a similar warning. Like the bit before Big Brother starts: *Some people may find the following procedure offensive and disturbing as it contains scenes of nudity, brutality and flashing images.*

For those who are mammogram virgins, let me explain. It's

a relatively simple procedure. They take your boob and squash it as flat as possible into a panini machine, or a similar piece of equipment, all the time twisting the breast, crushing it as the panini machine lid is closed and a ten ton weight of metal pushes down. You are instructed to hold onto the safety handles because during the procedure you will be contorted into the most impossible yoga positions while x-rays are taken of your boobs and armpits.

Once you are clamped into the afore-mentioned machine, a red danger signal will be illuminated and a skull-and-crossbones will light up. The medical staff will run away as quickly as possible outside the door, bolting it behind them. This is to prevent any highly toxic rays contaminating them during the x-ray process. As highly trained members of staff, their health and safety is paramount. Unfortunately you might be fucked, as there is no escape while you are imprisoned by your boob.

At this point there should be some kind of bloody announcement: *We recommend not inhaling the poisonous particles so please do not breathe at this time. Dimming the lights is common practice in hours of daylight, so you will be all alone in the dark. A short beep followed by re-entry of the panini machine operator and her pal will indicate this procedure is now complete. Once you have been released from the panini machine, do not be alarmed if you pass out. This is quite normal and you will come round again in a few moments. Do not attempt to speak to or distract the staff as this could lead to them choking on a chocolate or losing their Snapchat story. As you regain consciousness please pick up your bin sack of clothes and belongings and exit promptly. There is always a queue outside so your co-operation would be appreciated. Please be aware your gown is front fastening and will have a tendency to flap open. Women of a certain age take note... nobody wants to see your droopy old swingers. We hope you have enjoyed your mammogram experience and we look forward to welcoming you back in the near future.*

As my dear friend Ali Park once said, 'If you want to know what a mammogram feels like, open the fridge door, place your boob inside and slam the door shut.' Ouch! This is the twenty-first century... surely there has to be an easier way?

The Car Park

BACK IN THE CAR, I was surprised at how limited my movement was. As I tried to fasten my seatbelt the pain was intense. I had to take my arms out and just wear the belt round my waist; the slightest movement sent waves of pain down my arm and my chest. The small amount of anaesthetic I'd been given earlier had well and truly worn off, but that was the least of my problems.

It was then that Alan called me on my mobile. At last he had reception; he was just outside Aberdeen. He was excited about coming home and he talked quickly, the upbeat tone of his voice a stark contrast to my downbeat state of mind. He was desperate to hear about Molly and how I got on at my well woman appointment... how ironic. He fired a barrage of questions at me.

I tried to sound as normal as possible, terrified my voice would betray me. I hadn't had time to decide what to tell him and I certainly didn't want to say anything over the phone or when he was driving. He asked me if there was something wrong, and I remember telling him I had to go because I was trying to reverse out of a really tight space into busy traffic and I had to concentrate. Reversing into busy traffic didn't exactly make sense but it was the first thing that came into my head. I reassured him that everything was fine and that we couldn't wait to see him when he got home.

I hung up, took a deep breath, and stared at the deserted car park. I have no idea how long I stayed like that. But I knew I had to pull myself together, that it was no time for tears. I had to be strong. I was a mum, I was a wife, and my daughter and husband needed me. We are a very close family – we like doing things together, and it never feels right when one of us is not there.

The most important thing was to see Molly. To be a mum. I had to get back to normality, back to the safety of home, our happy space where none of this existed yet. Cancer had no place there. Alan would arrive in a couple of hours. We would pour a glass of wine or two or six. We would chat and laugh, it would be good to see each other again. I thought about all the times I had tucked Molly into her bed, cuddled up, and read a story together. We would laugh as Maggie, our toy poodle, would jump on the bed to snuggle up too, her little woolly tail wagging and bashing Molly on the nose.

Just one more night... tomorrow we would talk.

When Sharks Attack

THE BULL SHARK, THE TIGER shark, the great white shark. All different, all unpredictable, all capable of causing fatalities. They have a reputation as potential killers. So we fear them. The same can be said about cancer. There are many different types, all unpredictable, all capable of causing fatalities, and it has a reputation as a killer. So we fear it.

If telling Alan about my cancer diagnosis was hard, telling Molly was going to be horrendous. Having breast cancer only meant one thing to Molly. A fear that made perfect sense for an eleven-year-old girl who had never known the joy of having her grannies around. That's the thing about the disease, it can devastate families, robbing us of our precious loved ones. Both Alan's and my mother had died from breast cancer before Molly was born. It was very important to us to keep their memories alive so that Molly would know what wonderful women they were. She often asked us why she didn't have a granny, why cancer had taken them away from us, and as a young child she tried to make sense of it by writing this poem:

My granny is an angel, she lives up in the sky,
And cos I cannot see her, it makes me want to cry.

She also drew a picture of her grannies as angels flying in the sky with Robbie Burns. Random, but very patriotic. It made me wonder what was really going on in her head!

Talking about what goes on in your head, what the hell were the people who made those cancer adverts thinking about? The adverts that were being shown when I was diagnosed were appalling. I mean, for God's sake, who came up with the concept of a man standing all alone in a bleak deserted location, wearing only a hospital gown, with an even bleaker voice declaring 'cancer is a lonely place'. Oh bugger off! Nobody needs reminding, thank you. The messages were so depressing. Then Sir Alex Ferguson? Whilst I am sorry for what his family suffered, could anyone appear *more* gloomy? Every message they showed was just so damn negative, it was frightening. At least now they try to present the more positive message that life can still be enjoyable despite having cancer.

A lover with cancer is still a lover. Hey, that's great news, thanks for pointing that out. Who needs two boobs anyway? Your partner will still love you. Well that's a relief!

It seems to have almost gone too far the other way though, as two jolly bald girls are seen laughing and joking their way through chemo. I could have done with them in my chemo ward. Instead, nobody looked at each other, everyone lost, I presume, in their own 'lonely place'. Actually, it can be scary to look at each other. It's maybe an act of self-preservation, but you have to remind yourself that cancer is not contagious and your experience will not necessarily be the same as theirs. Even so, a passing nod to those around and a reassuring smile to the new patients was the most any of us seemed capable of.

It's funny how something you didn't really notice before suddenly becomes so prominent. It felt like every two minutes there was another cancer advert on TV. Cancer posters seemed to appear overnight on buses and buildings. All of a sudden, people were talking to me about fighting cancer, using language that described it as my 'cancer battle', which really jarred with me. I preferred to think of it as 'a healing journey' rather than a battle or a fight... that was way too scary for me. I could lose a fight.

Years earlier my mum had lost her little sister to cancer. Moyra lived in Zambia and, in the days before computers and mobiles, when an airmail letter would take up to two weeks to arrive, it made it all the harder for two sisters who were so close but living so far apart. I couldn't help but think about my own big sister. We were also very close, but she lived in Australia.

My fear of history repeating itself was palpable.

Mollywood

AS A MOTHER, MY MOST overwhelming fear about being diagnosed with cancer was not being around for my child. Obviously we had no idea how the journey was going to play out for me. We still had to wait for results to see if the cancer had spread anywhere else. All I knew was that I needed to get through it for Molly, for Alan, for all of us. Whatever the results said, I was determined and my thoughts became like a laser beam: sharp, focused, moving forward with only one end point... survival. My family was not being broken apart again by this disease. We were all affected by it, and we were all suffering because of it. I was extremely concerned about how Molly would handle it emotionally and I was terrified that she might feel she had to hide her true feelings or lock herself away. There was so much change happening already in her life, she was only eleven years old and she was so vulnerable. Alan and I just wanted to protect her, so we made a few simple rules:

It's ok to feel angry.
It's ok to feel scared.
It's ok to cry.
It's ok to laugh.
It's ok to forget all about this and do normal fun things.
We should always feel we could talk to each other.

No secrets, no hiding our emotions or whispering behind closed doors, as some people tried to do with us. I explained to them that shutting Molly out would only create more fear in her. I would tell her the truth and show her that it was perfectly acceptable to emote.

We lived as normally as we could and tried to forget about it till the final results came through. If the cancer had spread then there was no bloody point in being miserable yet. Time to fire up the happy hormones. I was good to myself. Until my chemo started I drank champagne, there was going to be plenty of time for that sobriety nonsense over the next year. Lots of humour, lots of laughter, no stress... those were our ideals and we tried hard to stick to them.

A week later the long-awaited biopsy results came through. I had cancer in the breast and lymph glands under my arm, but the cancer had not spread anywhere else. It was a massive relief.

As I mentioned earlier, I was fitted with a clip to keep a check on any changes in the breast. (I am already disassociating myself from it – *the* breast, no longer *my* breast.) Then I was mammogramed again. From that point on I asked no more questions about the cancer. I didn't need to know. I was doing this my way and I certainly did not need to know if it was aggressive or anything else. The less I knew, the less it could affect me mentally and I realised my mental state would play a massive part in my journey. Fortunately any concerns we had about Molly's emotional welfare were unfounded, and she expressed herself through writing. She summed up her feelings very well in a homework assignment, was encouraged by her teacher to give a speech to her class, and even started her own business: 'Mollywood Makes'!

Her coping mechanism combined her passions, hobbies and skills, which at that time mainly centred around make-up, skincare and making 'stuff'. After finding out that my immune system would be compromised during chemotherapy, and that a lot of pampering products were unsuitable during my treatment, Molly decided to do some research of her own. She decided that just because you have cancer, it is not a reason to stop caring for yourself. She went online to research natural beauty products and how to make them. She would then sit for hours and plan her range, using natural yoghurt, fruit, vegetables, honey and more. The internet was a great source of information for her; she watched copious demonstrations and listened to the wisdom of the makeup bloggers. She was forever ordering little plastic pots to put her products in and my fridge was crammed full of moisturisers, lip balms, body scrubs and so on. I have to say they were absolutely lovely and very good products. Unfortunately we had to tell her she couldn't actually sell them. But, not to be deterred, she took them to school, prepared a talk about her products and why she had made them, then let people try them. They proved to be very popular among friends and family, and everyone we knew that year received something from the wonderful and very professional range of 'Mollywood Makes'.

Maureen

IT WAS CHRISTMAS 1996 WHEN I was lucky enough to meet Maureen. At that time I didn't realise what an impact she was going to have on my life. I was thirty-one years old and had just started going out with her son Alan, who I was working with at the Pavilion Theatre in Glasgow. It was panto time and the production was *Cinderella* starring The Krankies – Janette as Buttons and Iain as the Baron. They were great fun to work with, full of nonsense and hilarious showbiz stories, and we had a lot of laughs on stage and in the pub after. Alan was a young twenty-four-year-old *foncy doncer*, and I was a slightly older but leggy Dandini. That was back in the days when females played principal boys wearing nothing more than a blouse, a waistcoat, fishnet tights and thigh length boots! Even the dancers wore more.

I actually have to thank Janette for making sure Alan's rather muscular physique, hairy chest and six pack were on display. He first caught my attention during the ball scene – she was dressed as Madonna, and performed a dance routine with him and another male dancer. As you can imagine, it involved a lot of innuendo, very little clothing and plenty of comedy faces, as at her height she only reached their waists. She danced and sang with the boys then turned upstage to catch my eye. I had to stand on the staircase throughout her routine and not laugh. Not easy when a pint-size pop princess pokes you with her oversized triangular boobs and makes suggestive one-liners under her breath, much to the amusement of everyone else.

My relationship with Alan began as fun and was based on laughter and friendship, which is also what Alan's family and friends provided in sack loads. Maureen and I hit it off from the beginning. Her straight talking and her sense of humour really appealed to me. I adored her. Whenever we were in Glasgow we spent time with her and Alan's dad David (who I also love dearly), because they were both great fun. Working in the theatre we did travel and tour around a lot, so time spent together was precious. His mother once commented on Alan's lifestyle, 'Aye very good son. You've got your town house for shagging and you come home to get fed.'

As time went on Maureen and David were a welcome part of our group, and a visit from them was always memorable. Once I offered to drive the pair down to York to visit Alan, who was working in the touring production of *Joseph and the Amazing Technicolour Dreamcoat* at the time. When I arrived at their house to pick them up they told me they'd be right out. Nothing prepared me for what happened next. The front door opened and out they came carrying a small table and bags. They flipped up the front seat and the pair of them climbed into the back of my car, putting the table on the floor between them. With much rustling of bags and paper, two crystal glasses were then produced and polished followed by a large glass ashtray. With their table laid, ice cubes clinking and drinks poured they were ready to leave. Thankfully they were both small as my car was only a three door Peugeot 205. It sounds mad and it was. I had expected one of them to sit in the front for the four-hour journey! However, despite sitting in the back, the chat never stopped and they were great company. Alan had said not to let them arrive tipsy... I thought he was joking.

Having a bar in a car was new to me, and after a few whiskies and only half way into the journey the inevitable happened – they needed a wee. With no services for miles they told me just to pull into a layby. David with his walking stick managed to hop over a fence and disappear into a field, but Maureen insisted she would just do it at the roadside. I thought I would cover her with my car door so the entire motorway did not see her squatting, but what I didn't know was that she had a bladder like a camel and without warning a river gushed out of her. I was standing trying to keep my canvas shoes out of the ever-deepening stream whilst holding the door open, and of course the more she laughed the more uncontrollable her flow was.

Finally we got on our way again and arrived in York. I parked up and went to meet Alan, who asked me if they had behaved and whether they had been drinking. He obviously knew what to expect. I told him they were as good as gold and that it had been a very entertaining journey. It was only as we walked back to the car I saw the back shelf was littered with miniatures. Daft buggers. It didn't take Alan long to see the funny side.

Now before I make them sound like a couple from *Shameless*, I have to say that nothing could be further from the truth. Maureen was very family orientated and so proud of her boys. It didn't matter how late you arrived for a visit she was always over the moon to see you. She offered that wonderful west coast hospitality, forever trying to feed you or give you something to drink. Then she would rush upstairs to wake David up, trying to entice him out of bed at some ungodly hour, 'C'moan David, get up. Want a wee prawn and a wonton, want a wee hauf? C'moan they're away tomorrow. You can sleep all day then.' She always managed to get him out of his bed and another impromptu party would start.

When Maureen was first diagnosed with breast cancer it was a terrible shock. We were working away a lot then so we didn't always see how much she was suffering. However, in true Maureen style she handled chemo and her mastectomy with courage and humour. Obviously there were some very dark times but that's not what she focused on. Her aim was always to make you feel ok, to make you laugh. Being bald meant the chance of new hair styles, and if she could do something to amuse people then she did. Wearing her wigs at jaunty angles was common practice.

Maureen was incredibly brave and recovered well, much to everyone's relief. Life returned to normal for another year or so and Maureen seemed fine. Then one day we were out for a drink together and she announced that she had found another lump.

The whole bloody journey was to repeat. The cancer was back. This time it was a lot more aggressive but that still didn't stop Maureen or break her strong spirit.

'Nothing like a good dose of the cancer to make me straighten oot and fly right.'

She used to tell a story, completely true, about a junior doctor in the hospital. He was quite nervous and as a result very serious. At one stage Maureen's lungs had filled with fluid and they needed to be drained. The young doctor arrived to examine her and asked if he could listen to her chest and back. She sat up on the side of the bed but as the doctor loosened her gown to sound her back her prosthesis flew out and landed on the floor. Squealing with laughter she bent down to pick it up, at the same time as he bent down to pick it up. At that moment his stethoscope got tangled in her wig and yanked it off. The poor young guy was so embarrassed he had to leave and let another doctor take over. She roared and laughed and she never let him forget it. She would re-enact the story for every visitor that came in, laughing hysterically. Even the young doctor managed to see the funny side eventually.

David and Maureen were never off the teletext constantly booking another holiday. Life was for living and they were living it to the full whilst she was fit enough to travel. Despite a double mastectomy Maureen posed topless for holiday photos on their apartment balcony, which David proudly framed and hung up at home. If she could accept her body then so could everyone else. At a family party she even allowed herself to be dressed up like a drag queen from *La Cage Aux Folles* in stocking cap, drag queen make-up, and a couple of nipples painted on her scars. With a pair of socks stuffed down her pants she danced into the room, determined to keep everyone entertained. Her incredible inner strength meant that she turned every challenge she was presented with into something positive.

Prosthesis, double mastectomy, mouth sores, severe pain, sickness, baldness. She dealt with it all. Sadly though not even Maureen's strong spirit and loving family were enough. The cancer travelled to her bones. This time the shark's bite was fatal... she was only sixty years old.

We said our final goodbye in the Prince and Princess of Wales Hospice surrounded by the people who loved her so much and who in turn she loved 'Oot their skin.'

It was June 2001, and our world had just lost its star turn. But even after she passed away she managed the last laugh... as each family member in turn kissed her goodbye, I was last in line. I bent down to hug her and kiss her cheek when her body let out an enormous sigh. I nearly jumped out of my skin and my language was choice. Apparently it was her lungs emptying, but I swear she did it deliberately, as her words rang in my ears, 'I told you Gillian, I love you oot your skin.'

* * *

WHEN I LOOK BACK NOW, I can't believe we only had four years together. Maureen was the kind of person that made you feel like you'd known her all your life. Everyone has so many stories about her. We talk about her constantly to Molly. They would have adored each other. Sometimes when I get the feeling: *Och Maureen, I haven't seen you for ages I wish you were here*, we are lucky enough to be able to put on a DVD and suddenly she is back in the room. We still cry with laughter at her antics, which reminds us how laughing usually led to Maureen wetting herself.

Her two sisters, Irene and Winnie, were on holiday in Spain with her, and one day they decided to have a refreshing beer with their lunch. Afterwards they decided to go for a bit of shopping. They were in a t-shirt shop and as they tried garments up against themselves, Winnie decided she liked Irene's better and was trying to convince Irene to take a different top so she could have that one. Maureen started to laugh and couldn't stop, and having had a lager at lunch she started to wee. The man in the shop went to get a mop wondering where the wet was coming from. Then he spotted Maureen, Winnie and Irene... 'Hey! No pishy pishy!' he shouted as he threw them out of his shop.

The first time we told Molly that story, she laughed so much that she bent over double and squealed as a dark patch spread down her trouser legs. It seems that Molly has been blessed with the same uncontrollable bladder as her granny. I guess the apple never falls far from the tree.

Doors to Manual

BY THE BEGINNING OF 1998 I had started to feel stuck in a rut. For the previous ten years, after graduating from the Royal Scottish Academy of Music and Drama in Glasgow, I had worked mainly in television, both at the BBC and at STV where I spent many years playing the character of Lynne McNeil in the Scottish soap opera *Take The High Road*. I was also lucky enough to work in lots of theatres around the country and have a successful radio voice-over career. But whether it was a pre-midlife crisis or just part of the grieving process, suddenly this wasn't enough. I seemed to be working in the same cities for the same companies and I needed to break free. I had only ever known the job of being an actress, and I realised there was a big unexplored world out there. I thought I would feel refreshed if I had a change of direction for a while. I was fortunate to get a job with British Airways as long-haul cabin crew operating out of Gatwick. We were known as the *Beach Fleet* as, with our contracts, we were lucky enough to only have to fly to the Caribbean, South America and Florida. It was a fantastic job, my office was the beach: white sand, turquoise water and stunning tropical gardens. The only decision I had to make was which bikini matched which sarong, a far cry from the thermals, dungarees and cagoule required whilst filming *Take the High Road*. I was also fulfilling another childhood fantasy of dressing up in an air hostess costume and clacking through the airport with my trolley case.

During my first flight to Tampa, Florida, I was allowed to sit in the flight deck. It was such a buzz and worth all the weeks of stress involved in the SEP training course. The aircraft was a DC10 and I was given the seat behind the captain, whilst a first officer and a flight engineer sat on the right. I could hardly contain my excitement during take-off. This had to be my best role yet. As the enthusiastic captain explained some of the controls to me, I started to fantasise about flying these 'big birds' (his description, not mine). As the explanations became more technical I found myself zoning out, and I definitely had my head in the clouds as I imagined myself, in that front seat, addressing the passengers:

'Good morning ladies and gentlemen, this is your captain speaking. Yes, it is a woman. Now for all you nervous fliers out there don't panic, the aircraft will actually be flying itself today, and once on the ground I am a dab hand at parking. The staff are always so pleased to see you, they actually save you a space and direct you to it. In fact, on arrival there's a wee man that waves his flags to welcome us in. Somebody ought to tell him it's dangerous to stand in front of the plane. The other good news is that there's no tricky reversing to worry about as the ground staff will push us back. Which is just as well, as I don't have a rear-view mirror up here. We are currently flying very high, and the outside temperature is really, really cold. As usual it's a beautiful day here on the flight deck, so I am faced with a difficult decision... should I wear my Raybans or my Guccis? Our routing today will take us over lots of countries, but as we will be above the clouds you won't be able to see anything. Just hope you people with the window seats didn't pay extra. We will be experiencing some light turbulence shortly. I never checked the weather forecast, but the first officer just told me to switch the seat belt sign on right now. Oops... wrong button. Don't know what that one was for. We would ask that for your safety and comfort you remain seated with your seatbelts fastened really tightly. Oxygen masks are probably going to drop down so make sure you grab one and I will try and find the switch to start the oxygen flow. Oh, apparently that's automatic too. Well I just hope there's not a power cut. If it's anything like the lightning storm yesterday, you are in for a treat. Och battered to hell we were. It was like being on the waltzers, but a hell of a lot more scary. Now, it's getting a bit busy up here, and I'm at risk of spilling my coffee on the controls, so I will hand you back to the cabin crew for further instructions...'

Suddenly I was jolted back to reality by a question from the captain and I wondered if he had noticed my glazed over expression. I realised I was probably more of a Lorraine Kelly than an Amelia Earhart, more interested in the captain's uniform than all the computer controls. Physics, geography, maths and weather are so not my thing!

I had the pleasure of working with some lovely crew, as well as some real bastards. Much like any job I guess. Apart from dealing with moaning and rudeness from a few passengers, which is inevitable on a long flight, especially when seated in the cramped cattle class that was called economy, the job felt like one long holiday.

I would work a flight outbound from the UK and could spend anything from a one night bullet trip to ten days relaxing down route. We were put up in fabulous hotels in the Bahamas, Cancun, Jamaica, Tobago, to name but a few. Alan and I enjoyed the perks of staff travel and I was able to take him on some of my longer trips – Christmas in the Caribbean and New Year in Nassau. We were living the dream. However, after about nineteen months, the icing was off the gingerbread. Despite being promoted, which meant I could choose where I worked on the aircraft, and the perks of the flight leftovers (duty free bags filled with bottles of wine, champagne and snacks) I was starting to get bored. The constant travelling abroad, then working a night flight and travelling back to wherever Alan was based in the UK, was exhausting. I was really missing the theatre. I was fed up with *herooties* on the flight, saying to me: 'Didn't you use to be an actress?' (A *herootie* means someone that recognises you from the TV. 'That's her oot of...'). I craved being around like-minded people. Also, it's worth pointing out that this was pre-internet and mobile phone. No facetiming friends in those days. A fax message was totally high-tech stuff. Anyone that knows me will probably laugh at that as I am more of a pen and paper girl and useless with technology, but I can at least make a phone call!

I'm not trying to sound ungrateful, but the job could be lonely. I was always working with different people, friendships were fleeting, and although I was used to that in the theatre, I really missed Alan. We wanted to be together, not living in different countries catching up when we could. I decided to hand in my notice and after a last trip to the Bahamas, I came home and went back to acting.

Funny how the universe knows what is best for you. Leaving the job meant we got to spend lots of precious time with family, and I was around to help and support Maureen and David when she became really ill. Maureen's passing made a huge impact on the whole family and poor Alan was heartbroken. He was so close to his mother, they had shared a very special bond. After her death it was like a little light went out in him.

He felt lost, and although he was working in a dream job in

the west end of London doing *Phantom of The Opera*, his grief was obvious. Everywhere was full of painful memories, and the grieving process was going to be slow and sore.

The Sound of Music

I DO LOVE MY BIG sister Jane. Although I am not so keen on her when she phones and wants to sing to me at eight in the morning! She has a very versatile voice and doesn't believe in restricting herself to singing in any particular key. She also has a large repertoire of material which she is keen to share, ranging from Verdi's *Speed Your Journey* to *Kumbaya*. You think she's about to hang up then the hills fill her heart with the sound of music and she will sing once more. *Eidleweiss* follows which then segues into *Flower of Scotland, Ye Banks and Braes* and even how far The Proclaimers had to walk, before arriving at the *Bonnie Banks of Loch Lomond*. The romantic scenery obviously affects her and it's time for the wedding section, starting with Billy Idol's *White Wedding* before stepping gaily into *Mairi's Wedding*. Finally she'll throw in a bit of Abba, Madonna, and The Bay City Rollers to complete the medley. All sung in a cockney accent. It sure makes for some unusual breakfast entertainment. I could blame the time difference, but let's just say that Australian wine is bloody strong!

My big sis is an amazing person. She is a super-duper success-ful, award-winning business woman who I and many others have immense respect for. I can't quite believe we came from the same parents (where did I go so wrong?) She is also a very generous and caring human being, and I am so proud to call her my sister. Jane has always looked out for me and protected me. She always seemed to know what to do, and even without asking she would be there for me. My brother-in-law Mark (her husband) is no different. I met him when I was fifteen years old, and although he and Jane were both at Edinburgh university, he would often come through to visit his friends in Dundee and sometimes even pick me up from school. He was like the big brother I never had and I adored him. I don't know why I am talking in the past tense, I still adore him, and through the years he has certainly got me out of some scrapes. I suppose it shouldn't have been a surprise that following Maureen's death, they were the people that helped us find a new focus.

In 2002 my sister asked if I would come to Australia and be a nanny for my young nieces Amy (four) and Ellie (two) whilst their own nanny was in America for a couple of months. We did not take much persuading. Alan and I knew it was just what we needed. I would go in the September and when Alan finished his contract in December he would fly out and join me. I rented out my flat in Glasgow and packed my bags.

It was such a special time. I loved being with Jane, Mark and the girls. I had missed them so much when they emigrated a couple of years before, and now we were all together living in a beautiful house, in a beautiful place, with a swimming pool, beaches and sunshine. I couldn't wait for Alan to join us. He had got a one year working visa, and although I was on a non-working tourist visa, I had some savings, so there were options to travel, and if we really loved Australia, there was no hurry to leave.

A couple of weeks before Alan arrived we went on holiday down to Margaret River. It was fantastic. The vineyards were an essential part of the itinerary and did not disappoint. There was also plenty of fun for the girls and even a bit of tennis. Now although I was a crazy tennis fan, Steffi Graff I was not. What possessed me to try and imitate her footwork I will never know. Two minutes into a simple hitting session with the kids and Mark, I fell over backwards. It felt like somebody had hit me with a cricket bat. There was a huge whacking noise, a sudden pain in my calf and I couldn't get up. Mark leapt over the net, knowing exactly what was wrong. I had ruptured my Achilles tendon. I won't bore you with the details but it required surgery, a stookie, wheelchair, physiotherapy, the works. Great timing for Alan arriving.

He was just so happy to be in Australia that nothing phased him. He seemed to be getting back to his old self, and we had such a brilliant time with Jane and Mark. We lived with them and when they were at work we would do jobs around the house. Shopping, cooking dinner, cleaning, helping with the girls and when they came home, we went to the pub for a couple of hours to give them family time. It was bliss. I was useless on crutches, but fortunately being confined to a wheelchair had its advantages... after the pub I could sleep on the ride home!

However, the happiness was short lived. Early in 2003 we heard that my mum had not been feeling very well and was short of breath. Over Christmas she was not her cheery self and phone-calls could be strained. Mixed reports were coming from the UK as to whether her health was deteriorating or not. It was unclear how serious her condition was, and I was unsure whether I should return to Scotland – a decision made harder by the fact I was still attending hospital and receiving intensive physiotherapy sessions for my Achilles injury, and my movement was very limited. Also my visa restrictions dictated how long I could stay in Australia and Alan had just started a new job singing with West Australian

Opera. Flying home was not going to be the easiest of journeys in those circumstances.

We had to wait weeks for Mum's test results and of course there was a backlog because the labs had been shut over Christmas and New Year. As January dragged on the results and biopsies were still coming back as inconclusive, however, a scan eventually revealed that there might be cancer. Just nobody was sure where... none of it made sense, and it was all very confusing.

At the start of February the news we had all dreaded came through. Mum had breast cancer. She had no lump, no outward physical signs. She had always taken good care of her health, especially after losing her little sister to cancer. Yet here we were again. The sharks were circling.

I had no choice. I was going home to be with my mum.

Louie

ARRIVING HOME TO THE SCOTTISH winter was a shock to the system, but not half the shock of seeing my mum lying in her hospital bed. How had this happened? When I last saw her in September she was a fit healthy lady full of plans to join us in Oz. We had talked frequently about Alan and I getting married and I used to joke with her about not needing a hat... unless it was a sunhat. No mother of the bride outfit required, a pair of flip flops and a summer dress would more than suffice.

Now my beautiful mum was lying there with an oxygen mask, drips and tubes everywhere. She was in a terrible way and I felt anger that nobody had told us how serious her condition was. Although to be fair, she had apparently been given her first dose of chemo three days before and was having a very bad reaction to it. Jane immediately booked a flight, leaving Alan and Mark in Australia with the children. When Jane arrived at the weekend Mum was starting to feel better. She told us how delighted she was to have 'her girls' home and she was determined she was going to be fine, she was going to beat cancer. Each day felt more optimistic as she went from strength to strength and talked very positively about getting better. She was enjoying hearing all our stories and having us near her.

We spent the next ten days together at the hospital. Despite her understandable fears, she put on a brave face, never complaining or self-pitying. On day eleven we were allowed to take her home for a short visit to see how she coped. We had prepared her bed-room and added a new tv with an integrated video player. She would be able to lie in bed and watch videos sent from Australia of her beloved grand-daughters.

With oxygen tank in tow we wheeled her out of the ward. All of us were on a high. Taking her home, even for a short while, felt like real progress. At that rate it wouldn't be long before she would be back on her feet. As we passed one of the hospital's boutique shops, she admired a very smart black suede waistcoat in the window and was delighted when Dad bought it for her. However, her visit home was not a success, she couldn't relax. The combination of being on oxygen and the pain she was in, especially during the car journey, meant she became extremely agitated. She was stressed and she needed to get back to the hospital. My sister and my dad drove her back, and I felt so guilty because I didn't go too, but I needed time out to process the situation. My earlier excitement was replaced by aching disap-pointment. I picked up the patterned paper bag that contained her new waistcoat and just held it close.

Louie, as she was affectionately known, was a very special lady. She always put other peoples' needs before her own, which could sometimes have a detrimental effect on her. Although some thought they could manipulate her for their own gain, her gentle nature and quiet demeanour belied her inner strength. Her family and close friends meant everything to her, and we all benefited from her encouragement and support. She was a great listener, not afraid to disagree if she felt something was wrong. We often sat down together over a bottle of wine and put the world to right... it was great therapy.

When we went to visit her the next day, she told us that we

had to get on with our own lives, that she would be fine and that Jane should go back to Australia, to her children and her job.

'Don't you worry about me. I've still got lots to do with my life, both with my current grandchildren and any future grand-offerings you girls care to present me with.'

Feeling much better, stronger and more confident about her recovery, she persuaded Jane to go back to Oz on the eighth of March. Four days later Mum was due to have her second round of chemo, but due to a sudden deterioration in her health it was postponed.

I was called to the hospital that morning at half past seven. They thought someone should be with her. That day I didn't leave. They provided me with a camp bed and I stayed by Mum's side. My dad looked drained, he'd had weeks of worry and I was very keen that he went home and kept himself busy. Hanging around a hospital was taking its toll on him.

There was fluid gathering at the heart and the doctors were sure there was another tumour near the lung. The cancer was metastatic. I had no idea what that meant. The doctors took my dad and I to a side room to explain, and they told us that we would have to decide whether to give permission to resuscitate. They advised us that it would not be a good idea. They informed us the cancer was very aggressive but would give us no indication of time left. This drove me insane. How could they not know? I couldn't accept that. Just tell us for God's sake! It was so shockingly unbelievable... the previous week she was going home and we were laughing and joking. My sister had just flown back to Oz.

My mum had obviously been told the same thing and when we went back into her room. She just said, 'So that's it then...'

It was the first time she looked defeated and resigned to whatever was going to happen. I had never felt anger like it. How dare they say that to her! How dare they just give up! Well I wasn't fucking giving up... if anyone could beat this she could.

After that bombshell she seemed to deteriorate rapidly. Rather than her giving up, I suspect it was more a case of her saving us from any more distress.

I persuaded my dad to go home and get some rest.

Mum was comforted by me staying with her and I filled the hours talking, reading to her or just watching her sleep. My brave and beautiful mum.

That night Mum woke up and called me over to her. It was 22:45 on the clock. She asked me to write down her last wishes. I had my Filofax with me and she recognised it as the one she had bought me the year before when they had been in Australia.

She requested two floral sprays of white lilies and that was all. One from me and Alan, and one from the rest of the family. No other flowers. How surreal to actually write that down. But I was prepared to do whatever she wanted.

She then said to me, 'Gilly, I so appreciate you being here.'

She held my hand and told me she loved me to bits. That was one of her last lucid moments and it was the last conversation we shared.

The next day, the fourteenth of March, was my mum and dad's wedding anniversary. How ironic. Dad came back to the hospital and I went home for a 'rest'. I actually had a shower and went for several brandies at the Monifieth Hotel.

Later that day I returned to the hospital and Dad reluctantly went home. Mum was now on a morphine driver, there was no response from her to any conversation. All through the night I sat beside her, watching as the morphine started to take its toll. I tried my best to comfort her as she was moaning and in obvious distress. She would start to climb out of bed but she was attached to drains and tubes and a catheter and I would calm her and tuck her up and keep talking to her. Throughout the night her morphine was increased and eventually she became peaceful.

The next day Mum remained peaceful but unresponsive all day. Dad had been there since early morning and I wouldn't leave her. By late afternoon I told him to go home, have a break and get some food.

I had read newspapers to her, done a crossword which I was useless at, hoping her frustration at listening to my incessant drivel would bring her back and she would wake up, give me the answers and tell me to wheesht. I wasn't going to give up on her, if she could still hear me.

At twenty past four that afternoon I was raking through her toilet bag in the bathroom telling her how nice her deodorant smelled, and that she would have to try this new shower gel when she felt up to it, when I felt a strong urge to go to her bedside. I had been thinking about popping out for a coffee and a firm 'no' appeared in my head. So strange.

I leaned over my sleeping mum and she breathed a couple of long peaceful breaths then finally the quietest softest breath that didn't come back out.

And that was it. My mum had slipped away, peacefully, unassuming, with no fuss, yet not without letting me know she was going.

It took me a few moments to realise what had just happened before I ran to the door and called the nurses who were stationed outside. The nurse was called Patsy. I will always remember that, as it was my nickname.

I was given a chair outside the fire exit, a black coffee and a cigarette and I tried to contact my dad. The poor man was not even home yet as he had stopped in at Aldi or somewhere equally mundane and normal for some shopping.

That is what struck me, all around were normal people doing normal things having a normal day... to me nothing would seem normal again.

I called Australia. Jane and Mark had friends over for dinner, and Alan was working. It felt so bizarre to hear normal sounds again – people laughing, drinking, happy. The shock was terrible for them and through the stunned silence of their friends I could hear my sister's hysteria as she tried to accept what I had just told her. Mark took the phone and asked if I was ok. Yes, strangely calm and functioning, I was fine. I was sounding normal, I had things to do.

When I went back in to see Mum she was serene. Patsy had taken flowers from the vase and placed pink and peach carnations round her head on the pillow.

I took Mum's hand and lay my head down on her now still chest. This wonderful, gentle human being, whom I adored, so still and peaceful. Love filled that room; it was her comforting me now. I could feel her energy all around, cocooning me. I stayed like that for an hour or so... there was no time, there was no noise, there was just pure love. Eventually I became aware of a feeling at my right shoulder that was moving higher towards the ceiling in the corner of the room. Pure loving energy. It was communicating with me although no words were spoken. I knew it was my mum, she was leaving. She was watching me clutch her now redundant body and she wanted to let me know. To say goodbye. Gradually the energy and feeling became weaker and the room was heavy and empty. As I looked at my mum she was empty too. Gone.

It was time for me to leave. The waiting and watching was over. It was time to join normal people doing normal things in the normal world. Without her. But I realised I would never be alone again. I had been touched by an angel, my mum.

Surreal Selfies

LET'S FACE IT, OFFERING CONDOLENCES can be awkward for some people. Some choose to avoid the bereaved altogether because they don't know what to say, and what they do say usually comes out wrong. Others feel obliged to visit and offer their guidance, whether you want it or not. The well-meaning 'grief police'.

'Best to get back to normal as soon as possible. You can't dwell on it.'

'She had a good life. She's in a better place.'

Really?

'Your mum wouldn't want you to be sad.'

That is true, but considering it had only been a matter of days and we hadn't even had the funeral yet, not to mention that we were waiting for Jane to come back from Oz, grieving was actually quite normal. I wanted to talk about my mum, but it was like nobody dared mention her. I felt like screaming, *It's ok to cry you know!* Talking about her made me feel close to her. In fact, the things people say and do in early days after a death can be quite irrational. I was asked by my family to write the eulogy for my mum, and after the funeral this old harridan of an aunt came up to me and said, 'Well, whoever wrote that certainly did not know Louie.' I didn't bother telling her it was me. Some folk are just not worth the effort.

Thankfully there are lots of others who are wonderful, kind, thoughtful and loyal. Who are there for you after the funeral when the grief police have long gone. I'm talking about the person who does something unexpected and most unusual, unconventional but heartfelt, and you can't help but adore them for it. We received a packet of photos that had been hand delivered through the letterbox. It was pictures from my mum's funeral. Pictures of the coffin, hearse, flowers and even ourselves standing beside them. Now I know it sounds weird and I can assure you, it was a new one on me. But I've kept the photos, although they are not something I look at regularly. Can you imagine...

'Come over for a drink and a bite to eat. Oh, and bring your photos.'

Obviously, we all deal with grief differently. They were actually taken by my mum's best friend Belinda, because someone had done it for her previously, and she had found great comfort in having pictures. The important thing was that the gesture was filled with caring and loving thoughts. In fact, you could say she was ahead of her time, a real trail blazer. The forerunner to selfies. Me and the hearse. Me and the coffin, It really is the last photo of Mum and me together. Sorry Belinda, you know we love you dearly as did my mum. But it's quite reassuring to know that I am not the only completely bonkers person on the planet.

The Grand Offering

As a child, the highlight of my Saturday night would be watching Olivia Newton John guest star on the Cliff Richard show. I loved her voice and her stunning good looks. As a teenager, nobody could have been a bigger fan of the musical *Grease* starring Olivia and my ultimate teen crush John Travolta. Wearing the iconic black spray-ons, off the shoulder top and high heel mules, casually dropping my cigarette butt, which was actually a rolled up bit of paper, and grinding it into the ground, I'd launch into *You're the One that I Want*. I had all the essential props of a hairbrush, a nightie, and a piece of tin foil... well, you can't perform *Hopelessly Devoted* without the reflection in the garden pond. I even had pink ladies in tow skipping round the playground to a chorus of 'Tell Me More, Tell Me More'. Oh man did we make that last note sound bad!

It was definitely those Australian *Summer Nights* I was missing, so it was inevitable that just a few weeks after my mum's funeral I found myself back in Oz. It was my dad who eventually persuaded me to go. I guess I just needed him to say that he was ok and it was alright to leave him. I was looking forward to seeing my big sis and the boys, not to mention the welcome distraction of my young nieces. Alan had wanted to do something really special for me as a welcome back surprise, so he organised tickets for an Olivia Newton John concert at the Burswood Casino in Perth. We are so rock and roll!

It was a real thrill to see her live, I nearly stopped breathing when she popped on a leather jacket, talked about the fabulous John Travolta and performed a short medley of Grease songs. It was the feel-good factor we all needed.

Life was starting to look up again. Alan was enjoying his job in the chorus of West Australian Opera and we decided we would like to make a fresh start in Australia. We began looking into immigration options. Despite Jane and Mark's incredible generosity, we decided it was time to get our own place and give them peace. We rented a lovely little two bed bungalow in a neighbouring suburb and we still saw them most days.

David (Alan's dad) came out for a few weeks holiday in the September, which was perfect timing as we had moved into our house the day before he arrived. I actually did the move myself as Alan was at work, lugging suitcases and boxes of possessions down a staircase very slowly. Amazing what you accumulate in a short time. Fortunately my Achilles was well on the mend thanks to a great physiotherapist.

It was the most beautiful little house, all on one level with an open plan kitchen and living room, ensuite bathroom, and outside dining area. We also had the luxury of going to Jane and Mark's posh pad whenever we wanted a swim in their pool. All was good and David was the perfect house guest. It was all very relaxed and chilled.

I guess you can sense things were about to change...

But not for the worse this time.

On the day before my thirty-eighth birthday I discovered I was pregnant. My swearing and loud exclamations even managed to wake David from his Bacardi induced slumbers (well, he was on holiday). I wasn't unhappy about it, more stunned.

I just couldn't believe it. Alan and I were Mr and Mrs careless, always hoping something would happen but it never had... until then. Crazy when you think I had been lifting heavy furniture and boxes totally unaware. Not to mention the copious amounts of wine that had been swallowed in previous weeks and, even worse, the cigarettes that had been puffed on. Not exactly the ideal preparation for pregnancy.

David was the first to know and he was over the moon for us. He spent the morning trying to convince me that Alan would be delighted. I had to wait till Alan got home from work to tell him and I felt apprehensive about how he would react, all sorts of worries had crept in to my hormonal head. Needless to say, Alan was beyond happy, ecstatic actually. It was our new beginning, our own little family. Both our mothers must have been hard at work arranging this grand offering! The next couple of months were filled with lots of celebrating, and my dad flew out in November to join us all and to escape the British winter.

Unfortunately, immigration didn't share our joy, and due to the imminent expiry of Alan's working visa, not to mention my age and the fact I was pregnant, we were not an attractive package. Ach well, their loss, and indeed the opera's, who tried to persuade immigration otherwise. But sadly it was a case of 'computer says no' and we had to return home to Scotland in mid-December. Just like Mary and Joseph we were looking for a place to stay as I had rented out my flat for another six months, not expecting to be back so soon. Fortunately, our really good friends Alan and Richard took us in and gave us their basement. Far more luxurious than a stable, it had a large double bedroom and bathroom, and was downstairs from the main house with its own back door. We could come and go as we pleased... a haven of peace. Funny how the universe looks after you, as we realise now it was right to come back and bring Molly up in Scotland amongst extended family and friends. Also our career opportunities in the arts were far better here. But God do we miss the sun!

Molly McNeill McKenzie appeared at ten to ten on the evening of the nineteenth of May 2004. It brought clarity and meaning to the phrase *a bundle of joy.* I was now a mum, experiencing for myself the magical bond that exists between a mother and her child, the invisible umbilical cord that pulls deep in your solar plexus. I felt like a lioness protecting her cub. When I think back to the last day in my mum's hospital room, I understand her just a little bit more. That unbreakable bond lives on.

Maggie

In 2005 we took Molly to Australia and spent Christmas at Jane and Mark's house in the beautiful suburb of Claremont. It was fantastic to be back. Christmas day on the beach with a new bucket and spade is a dream come true for any self-respecting toddler. Molly adored being with her big cousins Amy and Ellie, and they in turn taught her so much. She tried to copy them in so many ways, expanding her vocabulary, enjoying an al fresco shower just like them, and even wanting to start toilet training. With two big sisters much hilarity and high jinks were involved. It was lovely to watch them all together having such a happy time.

Alan and I also decided it was the right time to finally get married. So we did, in Parliament House Gardens, Perth, on the fourth of February 2006. It was a very small affair with no fuss. Our two dads, Jane and Mark, some Aussie friends and my best friend Petra with her twins William and Holly were all there. My bridesmaids were of course Amy, Ellie and Molly. It was thirty-eight degrees and Alan was wearing a kilt. Just as well he was a true Scotsman, as any available draughts were most welcome. We had an amazing reception in an outbuilding in Jane and Mark's garden, with a fabulous barbie and a swimming pool for anyone who needed to cool off. My Uncle Rob (Mum's wee brother) and his wife, Auntie Janet, happened to be in Perth on holiday and they joined us for our special day. It was lovely to have that wee link to my mum. I know she's never far away. We returned to the UK at the end of February 2006 officially as the three McKenzies.

Over the next few years our family grew in size, firstly with Ron the goldfish, a present from the dummy fairy that was chosen by Molly in exchange for her dummy. Mabel the house rabbit followed a few years later. Sadly Mabel was rather selective with her affections and obedience was strictly on her own terms. Saying that, I do have a lovely video of Molly and Mabel performing together – Molly practicing the Robert Burns poem *Tae a Moose* with Mabel being the moose!

Mabel was partial to naan bread and bananas and she understood certain words. At 'Nanabanana' she would hop down the stairs so quickly to get a piece that she couldn't stop herself smashing into the fruit and ending up wearing it as a bindi. When we ordered a takeaway Indian meal, she knew. She smelt the naan. One night she actually reached up and stole it before I could get it on the table, then went running across the room dragging a giant naan behind her. After that her free roaming days were curtailed to say the least.

We had originally hoped she would be a dog substitute as Molly longed for a dog but Alan was allergic to them. However, Molly was not put off and after doing some research she found out about hypoallergenic dogs. Month after month we were plagued with pictures and photos of toy poodle pups. She made a dog file with a wish list of characteristics. She knew how to break us! Finally we relented and we got our beloved Maggie, an adorable black toy poodle. She is so affectionate, delighted to be centre of attention, loves people and she loves going out, especially to the pub. But she prefers travelling everywhere in a bag! As a very small puppy she had a dog bag, and if that was not available then any handbag, sports bag, or carrier bag would do. She still has a bag, and it's non-negotiable.

They say some dogs can smell cancer and a couple of months before I was diagnosed, Maggie's behaviour changed. She never left my side. In bed she wouldn't let anyone lie beside me without her squeezing in between, and she took to lying over my chest, always curling up on top of my right breast. As the 'plum' inside my breast grew this became more uncomfortable. I would move her away, but she persisted. I am sure our incredible little dog was trying to tell me that something was wrong. Throughout my treatment Maggie stayed close to me, and it was very reassuring to cuddle up with her when I would come home, exhausted after a dose of chemo, and fall asleep. No wonder dogs are called mans' best friend. I think she saved my life.

The Breast Nurse

I'VE NEVER BEEN GOOD AT making decisions. I blame it on my star sign: a typical Libra. So I was almost quite relieved, when discussing my treatment options, to discover that actually 'options' was a surplus word. They were going to start with a course of chemo to try and shrink the plum, followed by mastectomy and removal of lymph glands, then finishing with radiotherapy. To be honest it didn't matter to me in what order it was served up. A three-course menu of delights with optional reconstruction to follow. I didn't have a clue what to expect. Like the first day in a job I was the new girl, apprehensive and a bit lost.

To support me through diagnosis, treatment and aftercare, they assigned me what I can only describe as a 'buddy'. This has to be the strangest job in the hospital. Your buddy is someone who holds your bra during an examination and books your next appointment. Oh, and during an examination she seems to be in charge of swishing the curtains, keeping them tightly shut and making it difficult for the doctor to get in or out. Why do they need to hold them closed, who are they hiding you from? Maybe it's so you don't get a draft whilst sitting there half naked.

My first experience of these strange people was of one standing in the room while I spoke to the doctor, quietly observing me like a minder, then silently fastening me back into my bra (which took me by surprise) after my examination, before escorting me down the corridor to reception to confirm my next appointment.

However you describe them – buddy, minder, governess, or indeed as I found out later, their official title of *breast nurse* – they are an essential part of the team. There are different types of breast nurse too. Fancy ones, plain ones, bossy ones, answer machine ones, even some friendly ones. To amuse myself in the waiting room I used to play 'spot the breast nurse'. I watched them as they wandered around the clinics, some in clacking heels and smart dresses, others more partial to comfortable slacks and a Scholl sandal, swishing and swiping their ID cards as they went about their business. All carrying files of paper, always checking lists, busy being busy. It was a different kind of busy from the doctors, who assumed an air of authority as they strode with purpose to their consulting room.

Breast nurses don't seem to belong to a room, they move between them, popping paper onto piles then picking it back up again, before moving off to peer at some more patients over another pile of paper. Sighing and talking to themselves.

Another job of the breast nurse is to lend you an information DVD about breast reconstruction. They are very strict with their DVD lending policy. You can only have it for a few days, as it is in high demand and they don't have enough copies. It reminded me of Blockbuster video shops and the fear of getting a fine for the late return of a film that was a new release. The DVD is presented by a consultant plastic surgeon, who is somewhat upstaged by his very large scarlet bow tie and matching pocket handkerchief. He likes to flare his eyes, maybe due to the bright lights or the strain of reading autocue. Occasionally he stumbles over his words, perhaps because he has an extremely posh accent and loose-fitting teeth. Undeterred he soldiers on and discusses a variety of options for reconstruction and the parts of the body they can use to create a new breast. Helping him explain is a very serious lady with a foreign accent. It was like watching the Queen deliver her Christmas message to the nation – very solemn and not given to frivolous displays of humour or personality.

I know it's not a laughing matter, but the seriousness of the presenters made me even more unsettled, filling me with dread. The DVD left me feeling a bit queasy. I was reminded that I was actually getting a breast cut off, and that if I wanted a new one I would have to sacrifice another part of my body. All the choices involved pros and cons and varied surgical and recovery times. I could feel another ostrich moment coming on...

Certain types of reconstruction were not an option for me due to my treatment plan. In other words, no simple silicone implants for me. Fantasies of having a newly constructed 'rack' that a twenty-five year old would be proud of were swiftly dispelled.

They were keen for me to make a decision before my first meeting with the plastic surgeon, although there was no pressure. I could have the procedure at any time in the future. Marvellous. No worries... as long as I remembered to bring the DVD back.

Before I offend every breast nurse on the planet, I would like to stress that it did not take long to realise what a fantastic job these highly specialised people do. The support and advice they provide during treatment and recovery is excellent, and I am hugely indebted to all the hard-working team that helped me. Thank you all.

The Bionic Man

I AM NOT SUGGESTING FOR a moment that there would ever be a good time to find out you had cancer, but it always seems to be the busiest of times in our household when things go wrong. My head was bursting with information overload regarding my own situation, yet I was still trying to focus on Molly's recovery, remembering to give her antibiotics at the correct times and alternating her pain relief meds up to six times a day. My brain was mush. I had to write everything down, terrified I would accidentally overdose her. It was also the start of the summer holidays, which meant that family were due to arrive the next day for their annual holiday in the west of Scotland. The Skrastins, the McNeills, the McKenzies, and the Birds, and I don't mean extra girlfriends! Every year we had a get together, where anything up to about sixteen of us would congregate at Crispie, a rented holiday house, in a remote but idyllic setting for a week, followed by the second week at Cameron House Lodges.

That year, however, Alan's tour dates meant he was away, and Molly was unable to travel as she had to stay near a hospital. But I still had to make sure my dad could get there as I was his designated driver. My *Big Bang Theory* kitchen planner was about to implode. This was a job for a grown-up person with good organisational skills who was able to manage and lead a team. Definitely not me then... help!

Bizarrely Mark ended up coming over on his own. Amy had to

study for exams and Ellie had dislocated her knee, which meant Jane had to stay in Oz with the girls. With everything going so well, it was shaping up nicely for a relaxed family holiday...

Oh, and Alan also managed to crash the car (perhaps he was reversing in busy traffic!) Actually, that's a bit of an exaggeration. It wasn't his fault and fortunately no one was hurt. Just a bump, which was fixable. But it was a rather unwelcome hassle, as we had to drive back and forward to Cameron House where my dad and Mark were staying at a lodge. If that sounds weird, remember it should have been my sister and the girls as well. We couldn't stay overnight because it wasn't dog-friendly.

We were also trying to keep my cancer diagnosis a secret. I had decided to let my dad enjoy his first week of holiday with everyone, before telling him or Mark. We would be seeing them at the lodge and I thought it would be better to talk face to face. He had been disappointed enough about not seeing Jane and the girls without any more bad news. There was also telling my sister to consider.

I wasn't sure how Dad would react... having lost his wife to breast cancer, how would he deal with his younger daughter being diagnosed with it? We are programmed to believe that there is a natural order to things. It's normal (there's that word again) to expect that the younger generation would outlive the older generation. However, as we all know this disease follows no rules. Neither does my father.

We call him the bionic man as he himself has been through an incredible journey. He has had brain surgery, and has electric wires in his head that somehow join onto a metal box implanted inside his chest. You can see the big thick cable through the thinning skin on his neck. This *was* meant to send electrical impulses to the brain to control essential tremor. He was actually one of the first patients to be a human guinea pig for the procedure.

The whole contraption is controlled by a battery operated exterior switch, and with a remote control held against his chest he can switch himself on. But it didn't work, even after it had been adjusted by hospital computers. The vibrations are uncomfortable and don't steady his hands. It turned out that the electrodes in his brain were put in the wrong position. His condition was made even worse, and the cowboy 'professor' who performed the operation has now, many years later, been struck off the medical register... at least in this country. Despite that he has set up as a brain surgeon in the States. Be warned, he is on the wanted list for messing up a lot of patients' lives.

My father was an artist and had used his hands for the intricate work involved in drawing, painting, jewellery making, and even tying his own fishing flies. Sadly the tremor made this impossible and he now can't even manage to hold a cup or write his name. But as they say, what doesn't kill you makes you stronger, and just as well. My dad is no stranger to cancer either. He has had treatment for leukaemia and still has occasional skin grafts for melanoma. Each time more cancer appears they chop it out, graft some skin from another body part and sew the new skin back on... he is starting to resemble a patchwork quilt. He's been through chemo a couple of times, though thankfully not with all the same side effects as I suffered. Still he bounces back. His daily pill count is scary. I am surprised you can't hear them all rattling around inside him when he shakes. As he says, if he tries to stir his coffee it becomes an instant cappuccino. I believe that his sense of humour keeps him strong.

Once he came through for Christmas to stay with us. Oh my

God. He had stitches in his arm from a recent skin graft and the nurse had not realised it was infected when she changed his dressing. Over the next week it developed into full blown poisoning. Vomiting so severe it was past the green bile stage, splashing up the bedroom walls, the smell of disinfectant thick in the air... we were at our wits end. My dad was seriously ill. A young NHS 24-hour doctor who came to the house suggested it was norovirus. I pointed out that if it was norovirus then we would all be ill by now and that he needed to get to hospital. Eventually the doctor agreed and an ambulance was called. Ten hours after arriving in casualty, thanks to the diligence of a smart junior doctor who eventually linked the infection in his arm to the sickness, Dad was finally admitted to hospital.

This resulted in a ten week admission, and at one point we didn't even know if he would manage to live alone again. He was so ill. Thankfully with some support in place he did. No disrespect Dad, but sometimes we do breathe a sigh of relief when we take you home to the east coast still in one piece. No wonder he says he doesn't like coming to Glasgow.

Dad's latest dalliance with cancer was bowel cancer. As a man in his mid-eighties the doctors were reluctant to operate, however they eventually agreed and successfully removed enough of the bowel to assure him they had cut out all the cancer. The doctors were delighted with the success of the operation. This was obviously great news and a huge relief, but it was life changing for him as it left him with a colostomy bag.

Although he managed to adjust and deal with it, I guess he had no choice. The mental scarring for Alan and myself, however, might take longer to heal! Obviously he couldn't change the bags by himself due to his tremor. At home this was managed by his team of carers, but Alan and I found ourselves in this most unenviable position when Dad came on holiday with us. No wonder they say nursing is a caring profession for dedicated people. I wholeheartedly agree, I think nurses are special. When you are not used to it, dealing with someone's personal hygiene – bathing them, cleaning wounds and reapplying colostomy bags – is definitely a challenge. I have huge respect for Alan taking this task on with me, as lots of people wouldn't. Especially helping someone who was so fond of curry. Root vegetables were off the menu. One bowl of my homemade lentil soup with a cup of coffee to follow could lead to complete devastation: explosion of the colostomy bag.

I have to say this was one time it was hard to see the funny side, but we all tried to. The most important thing was to preserve my dad's dignity as up till then he had been an extremely private man. He faced up to this new adjustment in his life with a positive attitude and just got on with it. 'It is what it is,' he said.

A few months after the first operation, discussions were afoot about performing a reversal, but again due to my father's advancing years they felt surgery might be too risky. Not for the bionic man. He underwent his reversal operation and I am delighted to say it was extremely successful. With what was left of his bowel stitched back together he was fully functioning again and no longer required a colostomy bag. Truly remarkable. His sense of humour, not to mention his dignity, was still intact.

His positive attitude to cancer is inspirational. Even when I told him about my own cancer diagnosis, I felt comfortable to cry in front of him and to admit that I was frightened. I found him to be a brilliant listener. He didn't overreact in fact he didn't say much at all – just quietly processed the information. It would be some time later before the "clangers" were dropped:

"Well I hope you last longer than your mother did."

"If you get really bad, you can get a blue badge."

Diplomacy is definitely not his strong point. However, I am so proud of my dad and the way he manages to stay so strong. He recently announced to us all that he fully intends to live to one hundred. After all, what else is there to do? He recovered so well from his surgery that he felt fit enough to visit Jane in Sydney for Christmas 2016. When my friend Lawrie asked how my dad was keeping he was stunned to hear that Ron was away to Sydney on holiday, 'He's away where? Oh for fucks sake, you're going to have to club him to death!' Dad thought this was hilarious.

As he enters his eighty-eighth year, I fully believe that he will reach one hundred. His positive attitude to cancer is inspirational. As I faced up to the tough times ahead of me, his experience and encouraging words filled me with confidence and I knew I would get through it. After all, I am the daughter of a bionic man!

Shooting Stars

NEWS TRAVELS FAST, BAD NEWS even faster. Letters and cards and heart-felt messages started to arrive at the house. I realised how lucky I am to have such supportive friends and family. However, it's strange that while there are plenty of funny or empowering cancer-related cards available online, I've never seen any in the shops. The 'get well soon' range doesn't really cover it, and nobody dared send me a humorous card. I would have laughed so much to get something that said, 'My oncologist is a lousy hairdresser'.

Instead, I received a collection of blank cards that people had opted to write their own message in. Most were brief, very positive, and full of good wishes, however it can feel like the nearest thing to reading your own obituary, especially when the inner drama queen surfaced in a couple of my friends as they described in detail how upset they were! To be fair to them, they were just showing how much they cared, and I would never have dared send a humorous card to anyone with cancer in the past. Now I think differently.

'I'm too sexy for my hair', or 'The hair and the spare'...

Ok I made that last one up, but I found these slogans strangely comforting, it made me feel accepted. Whether you find them funny or not, they do serve a purpose. Whilst some fill you with positivity others are a powerful reminder of the reality of cancer. 'Yes they are fake. The real ones tried to kill me,' I mean, would that not just encourage you to go home and check your boobs? The message that said the most to me was, 'I lost my boob not my sense of humour'.

As well as receiving cards, you receive people – lots of them, from the helpful to the hindrance, the cheery to the teary. One friend used to sob every time she saw me. Lawrie kindly decided he was moving in for a couple of days and would come back to stay every weekend... just in case it was terminal. Thankfully after a few visits he gave this up, as he had other things to do. Then there were the whisperers, the ones who couldn't actually say the word cancer out loud and whispered to Alan about me behind closed doors. And the planners, with promises of parties and prosecco or whatever I could taste when I felt up to it. And the stay away brigade, who try to avoid you at all times and wouldn't know what to say even if they saw you anyway. And finally, the ones who 'know what you are going through', even though they obviously don't!

Joking apart, our friends were brilliant and crazy, supporting us all in different ways. One friend Margherita, for example, took to wearing only headscarves or turbans. If I was going to lose my hair and cover my head then she would too! Whether it was as simple as teaching Molly to make a chocolate traybake, or taking her on fun days out, they rallied round. People were so kind.

My sister and her best friend Jacqui even planned an especially memorable surprise. Jacqui, her husband Dave, and their daughter Claire had rented a beautiful villa with a pool in the mountains near the Ronda Valley in Malaga, for their summer holidays. Jane and Jacqui arranged for us to fly out and join them for a few days. It was all organised and paid for and all we had to do was turn up. Five glorious days of fun, relaxation and sunshine, before flying home to start treatment. What an amazing present. Suddenly there was no time to think about chemo and what was ahead. We were so excited it was easy to forget our problems, as our minds were distracted with holiday highs and long 'to do' lists. When you don't have much time to plan it's amazing how quickly things come together. Getting my priorities right was essential... some last minute waxing, spray tan, nails, and sun cream were obviously top of the list, followed by euros, documentation, travel insurance, passports, boarding passes and transfers, and car rental. Then it was Mabel to the rabbit hotel, Maggie to my friend, keys left with neighbours, fish fed, bins out, and we were off.

It was absolutely joyous, everything you could wish for from a holiday. Jacqui and Dave were brilliant company and it was great to see Molly playing in the pool with Claire, laughing like a happy, carefree eleven-year-old should. All stress and worry forgotten.

One night, when it was pitch black, we took our sun loungers and lay by the pool staring up at the sky, which was filled with bright stars zipping about at great speed. It was so peaceful, so hypnotic. It was almost eerie. The vastness of outer space. Billions of stars, billions of planets, and us.

Now I realise it may start to sound like I was off my face, but I can assure you I wasn't. In fact, I only went along with it because Jacqui and Dave said we should. I mean, I have never paid much attention to what's up there before, I've never been that interested. It blows my mind when people start talking about galaxies, planets and distances in numbers that don't even exist. But this was awesome. I was totally mesmerised, immersed in the moment. As a child I was told that if I wished on a star, my wish would come true. I felt myself being pulled up and I was floating amongst them, so I made a wish. Then all of a sudden I heard a shuffling movement beside me. Something brushed against my face and pulled at my hair. I knew it wasn't the others messing about. They were still lying on their sun loungers at the far end of the pool. What was out there, lurking in the darkness? My imagination made up what it couldn't see... I certainly wasn't going to hang around to find out. The magic was broken as I screamed and bolted back to the house, moving faster than any shooting star, still secretly hoping my wish had managed to catch one.

What the FEC?

AFTER ALL THAT STAR GAZING it was back to earth with a bump. On Wednesday the twenty-second of July I had my first meeting with the oncology team to discuss my forthcoming chemo. The preparation for chemotherapy was far more involved than I expected. A thorough MOT is required. I think I visited every hospital in Glasgow in the process. I had bone scans, x-rays, a heart scan, blood tests... all just to ensure I was fit enough to withstand being pumped full of poisonous chemicals. Of course, after each procedure there is a wait until the results are processed.

I was grateful to have a lovely caring doctor, Dr Judy, who talked me through what to expect over the next few months. She explained the drugs that would be involved: Fluorouracil (5fu), Epirubicin, Cyclophosphamide, followed by steroid tablets and Docetaxil, or Taxotere as it's apparently sometimes called, which make up FEC-T chemotherapy.

She also explained that chemotherapy would be given in the day unit by a chemo nurse, and that the day before a phlebotomist would take a blood sample, which would be checked by a doctor to make sure I was well enough, before they instructed the pharmacy to prepare the chemo.

Anti-sickness drugs would be given before they started and my chemo would be administered through a cannula in my hand. It's weird but that is when it seemed to hit me, and my stomach was churning with nerves. I knew I was going to suffer but I couldn't imagine what it would feel like.

Dr Judy explained that the chemo would consist of several cycles over several months, each cycle of FEC-T taking twenty-one days. It would be divided into two parts, starting with three cycles of FEC followed by three cycles of docetaxel and steroids. She also warned me that by my second dose of chemo I wouldn't have a hair on my body.

It's just as well they give information sheets away with you, as the list of drug names made me feel as if I was listening to a foreign language. I didn't want to read about it though, as long as they knew what they were doing. They were in charge and I was just along for the ride. By the time she went through all the potential side effects I was on a damage limitation exercise again and switched to selective hearing. Some people need to know everything, I don't.

I did try to listen carefully to what she was telling me but eventually I zoned out. Still, that's better than passing out! Too much information leads me to protective mental shutdown (PMS). I would find it all out when it happened...

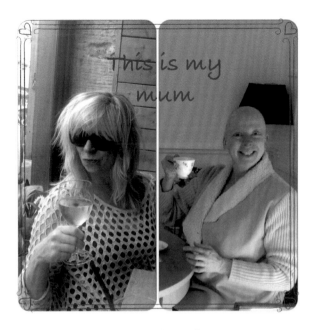

A collage by Molly.

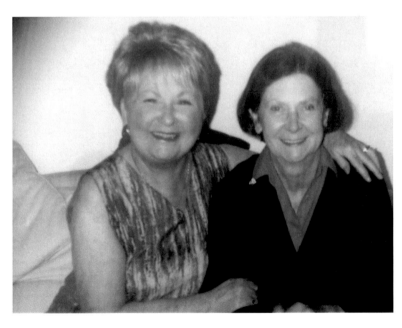

Maureen & Louie.

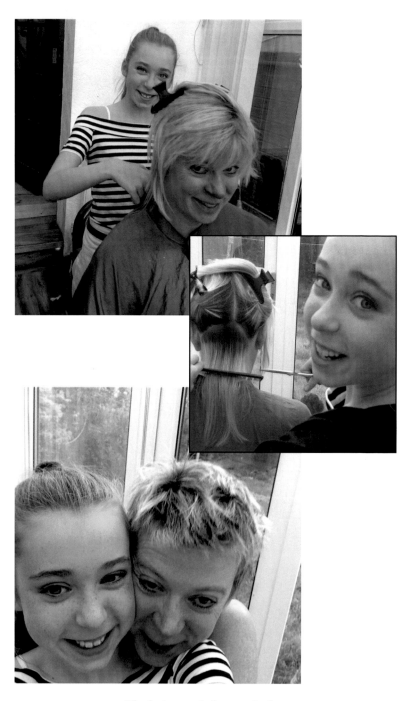

The haircut - before and after.

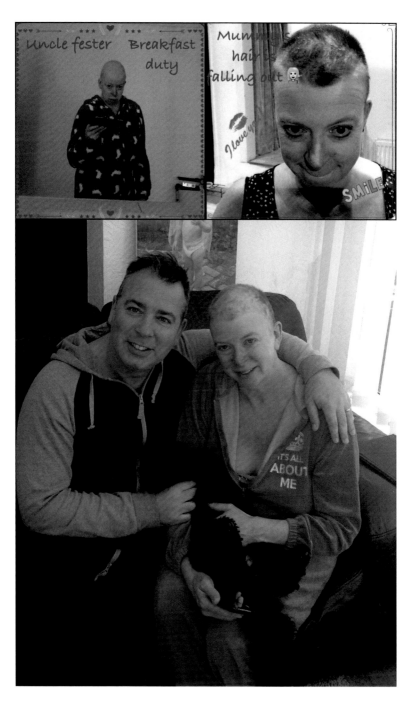

The hair coming out.

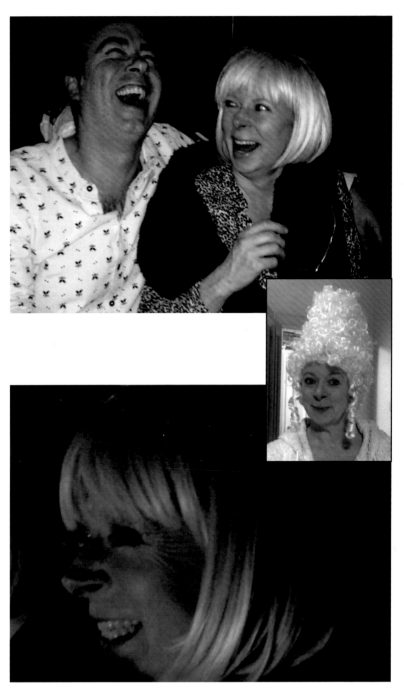

The wee peroxide bob (and a different wig!)
Bottom image taken at my 50th birthday party.

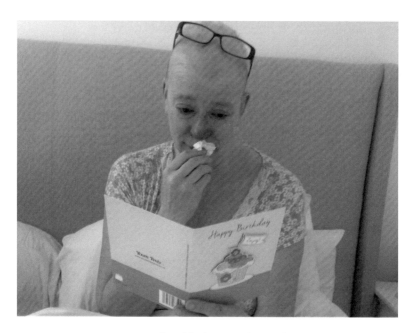

My 50th with those 'safe' cards.

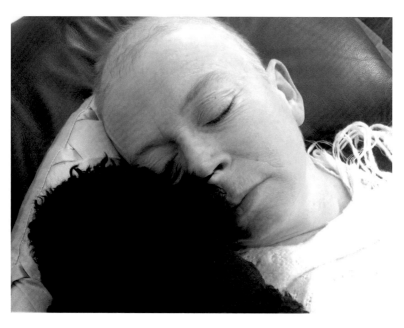

After a dose of chemo with Maggie.

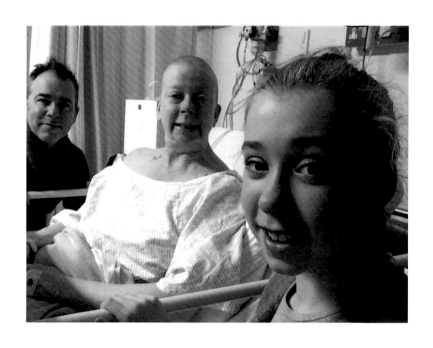

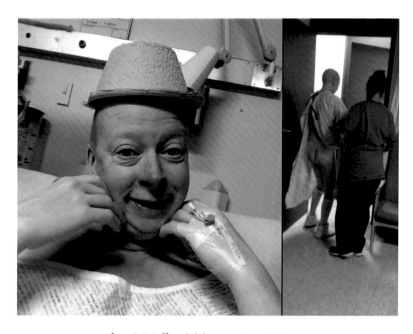

Alan & Molly visiting post-mastectomy
(and those big white see through pants!)

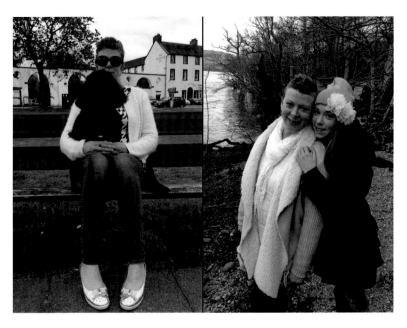

'Hey missus, you've goat the the same hair as yer dug!'
(Unflattering stages of hair regrowth.)

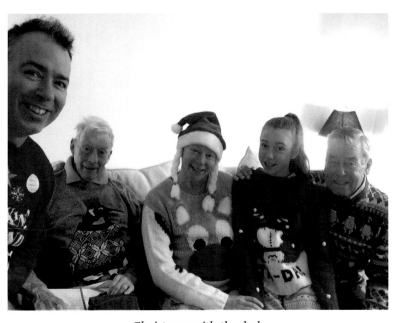

Christmas with the dads

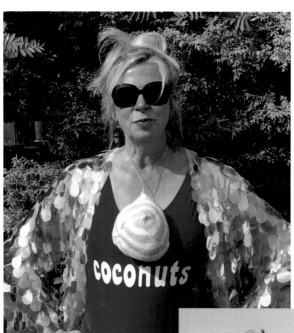

Petra's knitted knocker
(secure them by tying
down)

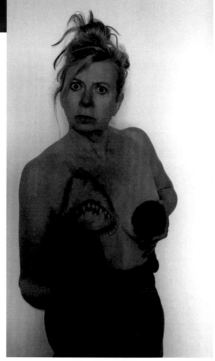

My shark bite
(beware of falling coconuts)

Discretion and Dignity

BUSINESS AS USUAL, IT WAS off for a heart scan followed by a spot of wig shopping. Hey, my life just kept getting better and better! With my list of wig suppliers and my NHS wig voucher I was all ready, but where do you start? I hadn't realised that there were so many places to choose from, all offering a personal and professional service and strictly on an appointment only basis.

I had imagined just popping in and trying one on, like going to a department store to buy a hat. The salons all had silly names like *Parrucche*, *L.A. Hair* and *Judy Plum*. Maybe that was a sign... my oncologist was called Judy and I had a lump called Plum. With an average waiting time of two to three days, I decided that whoever could take me first would be where I would start. I didn't know if they all carried the same stock or offered the same level of customer care, or if it would be just like a Primark fitting room – take in six items and try them on whilst a bored assistant asks if you want any of them, then tells you how fabulous you would look in that Mohican.

After phoning around I felt like I was about to get involved in some seedy strip joints as hushed voices informed me that discretion was the name of the game. Private rooms were available. An image of big burly bouncers and dimly lit basements sprung to mind.

That was until I arrived at the shop, which was actually located in a massive multi-purpose building opposite a busy railway station, complete with taxi rank and bus stop outside. Swarms of shoppers jostled me as I squeezed through the smokers loitering in the doorway then tried to peer at the list of businesses attached to the intercom.

Eventually I found who I was looking for after rummaging through my bag to get my reading specs. It was then I realised I already had a pair on my head, whose sole purpose seemed to be to hold my hair back. What did we all do before ninety-nine pence readers?

The buzzer was so loud that everyone turned around to look, and I quietly said my name, 'Hi, it's Gillian McKenzie for my appointment.'

'Who?' came back the crackly and over amplified response.

'Gillian McKenzie.'

'You'll have to shout. I can't hear you for the traffic noise.'

'I've got an appointment, it's Gillian McKenzie.'

'Are you here for a wig?'

Well, by now I had the full attention of the bus stop. Suppressed sniggering from the smokers was causing me to overheat as an embarrassed flush rose up, making my scalp prickle.

'Em, could you just buzz me in please?'

'Yes dear, now who did you say you were?'

To which the entire bus queue joined in unison, 'Gillian McKenzie.'

Totally mortified I was finally buzzed in alongside a group of office workers returning from lunch, as well as Alan and Molly, who had just arrived oblivious to what had taken place as they had been parking the car.

After requesting the fourth floor, which incidentally only had the wig shop on it, we got out of a very overcrowded lift. Ignoring the nudging and smirking and avoiding any eye contact with the smelly smokers who looked like they were going to self-combust if they had to contain their laughter any longer, we arrived at the shop. Another bell to ring, before I was pulled in quickly, the door hastily shut behind me and the blind pulled down.

'We pride ourselves on our discretion. Discretion and dignity for all our customers,' announced the shop assistant.

I believe the shop is no longer trading... I can't think why.

On display in reception were an array of wigs in many styles and colours, but there was no time to loiter as we were ushered into our tiny and overcrowded private room. Four humans, one dog in a bag, a chair and a mirror. The room was stacked high with hair-dressing equipment and wig boxes. The assistant scurried around her Aladdin's cave, up and down a small ladder, opening boxes, in search of the right wig. They try to match them as closely to your own hair length and colour as possible. These wigs are amazing, no cheap shite here! They are so well made that they even have what looks like a scalp showing through the parting. Some have highlights and all can be cut and styled to your liking. My only criticism would be that they are too perfect. Ideal for a woman who loves her blow dry, and a 'just left the hairdresser' look, but I am more your shabby chic kinda girl. Over styled hair just doesn't suit me.

Now, I have to say that the wig voucher they issue you with is another brilliant scheme. It saves you a fortune as, needless to say, these wigs are not cheap. Some run into three figures, maybe even more. Mine cost me absolutely nothing. I also opted to buy a stand, a brush, and specialist shampoo/conditioning shine treatment (which prevents it from going dull).

I was so glad to have Alan and Molly there to give me advice I could trust, and to offer words of encouragement or indeed bring some humour to the situation. It's a very strange experience, seeing yourself in a wig, and imagining having to wear it outside in real life. Totally different from the novelty of fancy dress or playing a character. The experience in the lift was playing on my mind. Would everyone stare at me? The hair just looked ridiculous and false on me. I didn't want to have to wear a wig. I found trying it on to be a very upsetting experience, despite the care and attention of the assistant and my family's reassurance.

I had no idea how sensitive and vulnerable I would feel without hair. Although I was still sitting there with all my hair intact underneath the stocking cap and wig, I think it was another moment of realisation about what was still to come.

Alan and Molly convinced me to order the wig. They thought it was lovely, but they didn't have to wear it. Even after getting home it lay in its box for quite a while, I mean days, before I would even look at it, let alone try it on. It may seem as if I was behaving like a spoilt child, but I wasn't being ungrateful, more just struggling to accept the situation. It made matters worse when I eventually put the wig on, and all I could think of was that I looked like the transgender boxing promoter Kellie Maloney. The relationship between me and the wig was going to take time.

Of course, if wigs are not your thing then there are a whole range of scarves and turbans, even workshops on scarf tying. Molly freaked at seeing me in a turban, but she wasn't the only one. I looked like I belonged in a French and Saunders sketch.

'You look like you've got cancer... like you're ill Mum, I hate it. I would rather see you bald than wearing that.'

I knew exactly what she meant. It was suggested to me that I could pin a large piece of costume jewellery on the front of my turban, such as a fancy brooch. Very *Sunset Boulevard*. Sadly I looked more like Hilda Ogden than Norma Desmond.

For me it was definitely going to have to be a wig.

Uncle Fester

Where, oh where is ma lovely hair...
It's not on the pillow, it's not on the flair.
When I went to bed, it was definitely there,
I woke up this morning, my head was all bare.

My transition from Goldie Hawn to Uncle Fester was remarkably quick and matched exactly what Dr Judy had predicted. By my second cycle of chemo I was bald. I made up a daft wee rhyme to say to Molly to make her laugh. It didn't matter how silly the words were, if it lifted my mood and made my child smile then it had served its purpose. Molly enjoyed making up further verses, and it really seemed to help her. I wrote a daft poem to Maureen when she first started to lose her hair; David still has the card it was written in because it used to make her laugh.

In order for this stage to be a slightly less traumatic experience for everyone, my fab friend and hairdresser Tracey suggested that I should start cutting my hair short in the days leading up to chemotherapy, so the sudden loss of my hair would not be so shocking.

The day before I was due to start chemo I got my heart scan results, which were obviously fine as chemo was still scheduled to go ahead. So next on the agenda was the haircut. That afternoon we went via the pub before picking Molly up from school, a bit of Dutch courage was needed before the big snip. Alan kept me topped up with large glasses of white wine in his role as barman and driver. Later that afternoon Tracey came to the house and gave me a rather fetching pixie cut. I had asked Molly if she would do the first big chop. Molly did a brilliant job even though she was so nervous, and somehow being involved with the hair cutting helped her to accept things.

I have to say I loved the pixie cut, and I wished I had done it earlier. Unfortunately the rather fetching new look was not to last. Within a week Tracey was back, clippers in hand, to perform a rather unflattering number one cut, followed a few days later by a brutal buzz cut. I think even Tracey found it hard, I was her friend and although she kept her emotions in check around us I could tell it was affecting her. I looked like Action Man with the wee bit of fuzz on top of my head, and I realised that I needed to find a more arty range of clothing to soften my appearance.

My pillow was covered with a soft down each morning, and I was developing a bald patch that resembled the worn bit on the back of a new born baby's head. My settee looked like a cat had been lying on it. There were more tufts of hair lying about the floor than in Pampered Paws dog grooming salon.

Whether I liked it or not, I needed to start getting acquainted with my wig. I was shortly going to need it. Maybe giving it a name would help. Any name would do, although definitely not Kellie...

I eventually decided that the wig looked like a cross between Agnetha from Abba's hair and Olivia Newton John's, which made me feel slightly better, and I was ready to give the wig a go. I did wear it to start with but I still didn't like myself in it. I was so self-conscious. It felt like big statement hair, although I had no idea what I was meant to be saying!

I even wore it to a wedding. However, the torturous combination of chemo two days earlier, high heels, Spanx pants, no alcohol, and massive amounts of hair that was hot, itchy, and stuck to the sequins on my dress, drove me bonkers.

I couldn't wear it up in case the mesh bits showed, and if I wore a jumper it stuck to it. Static caused it to radiate electric shocks to everyone. Trying to dog walk with Maggie on a windy day, in fact on any day, was a nightmare. All that hair whipping round my face, in my mouth, blinding me as I bent to pick up a poo... and on top of that I was terrified it was going to blow off.

I made the mistake of wearing it once to a parents' night at Molly's new school. As I sat in the overheated classroom I could feel the warmth rising, but wearing a wig meant there was no escape for all that hot air that was building up underneath it. I went through various shades of red, scarlet and finally beetroot before the sweat started to pour down my face, taking with it the foundation and eyeliner in long dripping streaks. I looked like a smudged face-painting of a tiger, all white, orange and black stripes. It was a first meeting with the teacher so I didn't feel I could just take my wig off. I sat there trying to pretend nothing was happening. What a great first impression to make!

After several failed attempts to tame the beast by cutting bits, pinning bits, wearing a hat over it, it was definitely time for a change. By that time I had amassed quite a collection of hand-me-down wigs from caring friends. Some were really not very suitable for everyday wear. Apart from the pile of pink wigs I was given, there were also some rather interesting alternatives. David had given me Maureen's old wigs, ignoring the fact that they had been played with so much and were matted and stank of mothballs, not to mention the slightly dated style. Let's just say it was a lovely gesture. Belinda, who can always find something unusual, sent me a range of wigs that her big sister had used when she had breast cancer – beautiful long brunette and strawberry blonde ones, now a great addition to our dressing up box, providing hours of fun when we have a party. But the best one she sent was what I can only describe as a monk's hairstyle. Her sister Sue lived in Hong Kong, where it could get very hot and humid, and the smart locals had come up with a brilliant alternative to a full wig. It was a circlet of hair you wore round your bald head, which you could then put a sunhat on top of, and it would look like short hair sticking out. It was hilarious. Unfortunately, the hair reminded me of the wiry, nasty stuff that used to be on my dolly in the 1960s. This definitely wasn't a look for Glasgow, but jeez did we have a laugh with that wig. I kept trying various styles, colours and looks to see if any would be a suitable replacement. Eventually Molly had to come and speak to me.

'Please Mum, don't keep appearing at school in a different wig, nobody knows you are bald and I don't want people to laugh at you.'

My poor little girl, I had been so focused on me and my wigs that I hadn't thought about her trying to fit in to a new school and make new friends. Obviously she didn't want anything to make her appear different from the others. She especially couldn't bear the thought of me being the butt of playground jokes. The new girl whose mum was a weirdo... I went back to wearing my proper long wig for school.

When I was well into my chemo the steroids were taking their toll and bloating my face. I had no eyebrows or eyelashes and I needed to wear a soft woolly hat for my over-sensitive scalp. I was desperate to find something that would detract from this.

I finally found it. I ditched the long locks in favour of a very lightweight peroxide bob that I bought from the party shop. I never looked back... cheap as chips, it was bold as brass, loud and proud. Molly and Alan loved it. A mother in the playground who had seen me previously with long hair stopped to tell me that she loved my new hairstyle. Wow!

When the wind blew you could see the crochet skull cap underneath, but I didn't care. It fitted like a glove, it was comfortable, light and easy to wear. That little wig saw me through it all. It washed like a dream, and was the best £9.99 I ever spent. As the man in the shop told me at the time, 'You cannae argue with a tenner hen.'

I learnt to enjoy wearing my wig, and there were lots of positives too. The very handy thing about a wig is that you never have a bad hair day. I loved the fact that I would always know how my hair would look for a night out. It saved so much time and stress, and Alan would have it all beautifully styled and ready to pop on after I was out the shower.

Just goes to show, you cannae argue with a tenner.

FEC Me

NOTHING CAN PREPARE YOU FOR chemo, it's just something you have to get on with. I know some people take vitamins and supplements or try special diets and wear ice helmets to prevent hair loss, but I didn't go down any of those routes. For me it was giving the cancer too much importance, too much attention, and the hair loss was inevitable in my case anyway. I did, however, undergo one major lifestyle change during my treatment – I gave up alcohol. Which, as anyone who knows me would recognise, was a significant sacrifice (I didn't get the nickname Patsy for nothing). So much so that Alan also gave up the booze to support me. What a guy. As it turned out, the last thing I could stand would be alcohol on top of chemo, so it was probably much easier for me than for him. However, he didn't complain once. I wonder if I would have been so strong-willed had it been the other way around.

I had my first chemotherapy on the thirtieth of July 2015, and I was so nervous beforehand. The worst thing is not knowing what's going to happen, fully aware that whatever they're doing will result in some pretty nasty side effects. Thankfully Alan was allowed to stay with me during my first treatment, which was hugely reassuring.

After they took my bloods it was a case of sitting in the waiting area until the pharmacy had prepared my treatment and we were called through to the unit. I was quite content to wait. My stomach was churning, and Alan was trying his hardest to make small talk that I wasn't really hearing. Finally it was my turn. We entered a ward with six stations, five of them occupied by men and woman wired up to machines and drips. Some sleeping, some eating, some reading, all in isolation and oblivious to everyone else. I stared at each one as I passed, wondering if I was about to have the same thing done to me.

My chair was right at the end next to a window, which looked out onto a grey wall and a tiny courtyard full of stones and a multitude of old cigarette ends. With no obvious access nobody could get out there, so where did the cigarette ends come from? That would occupy my mind for a while. What a dreary outlook for a chemo ward. Such a missed opportunity for something beautiful to fill the space. A pond or a plant perhaps, or even a trompe l'oeil of a garden scene, anything but bare concrete and old fags.

'Admiring the view? Lovely isn't it,' said a very sarcastic nurse as she approached. 'I'll just pop you onto the electric chair, no pun intended, and we can get started.'

Could she read my mind? That was exactly how I felt – like I was waiting for the electric chair!

She first showed me how to get in and out of the chair without injury, which was trickier than it sounds. It was one of those high-tech objects that did everything, including tripping you up. She provided lots of pillows and a table, more pillows for my arm, and a control panel for the chair, which I was shown how to work to achieve maximum comfort. From that point on make sure your husband does not have the remote control, as he will be tempted to play with it. One minute I was sitting comfortably, the next I was whisked backwards, legs akimbo, staring at the ceiling. Not for the first time... oh memories!

That's not the only gadget in the unit. Hidden behind beams in the ceiling, soft colour lighting goes through its automatic cycle. Now every time I see colour-changing lights it reminds me of the chemo unit. Finally a small radio set to extremely low tries to give an air of relaxation.

The nurse then brought me a basin of lovely warm water to soak my hand. Not quite the Carrick Spa, but so far so good I thought. Although I definitely had the feeling of a calm before the storm. The warm water dilates the veins, making the insertion of a canula easier. Not a problem for me as I was blessed with big fat juicy ones, a junkie's dream. Although by the end of several chemo treatments I became like a punctured balloon, or a human pin cushion, and my veins were a shadow of their former glory. Over time the insertion of the canula became a difficult and uncomfortable process.

I was given anti-sickness drugs before the nurse started administering the chemo. Then I got my first big fright as a trolley was wheeled towards me and I spotted them. Three ginormous syringes, panto sized in fact, each about a foot long, filled with a bright red fluid. Fec me I thought... and they did!

Two nurses start ripping open sealed bags of clear fluids to hang on my drip. They ran through a thorough check list, double checking identity, personal details, and medication checks. They can't risk a mistake. It's at this point you feel like shouting, 'No, that's not me, they must be for someone else.' Maybe that's why they allow a partner at the first session. To make sure you don't bugger off and hide in the toilets.

I cannot praise the work of the medical staff highly enough. They were brilliant, so patient and caring and cheerful. No matter how busy they were, they remained calm and outwardly happy.

Which was so important. A nurse had to sit beside me and slowly inject the red fluid (epirubicin) and the 5fu into my vein whilst a drip infusion flushed them through. Each syringe took about ten minutes to put in. I also got the cyclophosphamide as a drip infusion, which took about thirty minutes.

During treatment I was monitored very carefully and told to report any discomfort or changes. It's a strange thing, you sit there just waiting to feel something, wondering what it's going to do to you. I was shaking, not knowing what would happen next. Nothing did... just incredibly cold liquid going into my vein, which is a bit bizarre, I guess.

Thankfully I very rarely had a problem whilst chemo was being administered, odd issues with the canula perhaps, and once it leaked which was painful and stinging. I didn't report it at the time and suffered later when my hand swelled up. Luckily an eagle-eyed nurse spotted it and gave me a ticking off for not pressing my call bell. Sometimes I would get very hot or get a strange taste in my mouth, but there was nothing serious and the nurses were always on hand to check or adjust the drip speed.

I was surprised at how quick the actual treatment time was. I thought it might be hours. Although sometimes it was much longer depending on pharmacy and waiting times for chairs.

Something I was astounded by as I became a regular in the unit was the amount of complaining done by patients and their families, usually about how long they had to wait. They could even be quite abusive to the overworked staff. This used to drive me mental. Why couldn't they be grateful for their treatment? The staff were working to full capacity. When I heard them kicking off I felt like saying to them, 'Do you have something more important to do? Where else do you have to be that warrants this rudeness and impatience?' Some people just need to stop and appreciate how much they are given for free. The Beatson provide a fantastic service that is stretched to the limit.

Anyway, rant over. For now.

My first treatment complete, they sent me home with more anti-sickness drugs and some other meds, and a ton of new information to read. And that was it. First one down.

Red Card

THE FIRST WEEK AFTER CHEMO usually started well enough, I would just be extremely tired. By the second week all sorts of nasties would creep in and I would feel like crap as my white blood cell count dropped and my immunity lowered. This would sometimes result in hospital stays due to infections related to neutropenia. I think that's what they called it anyway... why am I even trying to use all these big names?

It was hard to get used to reporting what seemed like the most minor of ailments. The nurses were so busy, always rushed off their feet, and I was supposed to annoy them with something as trivial as a sore finger or a headache.

I was always getting into trouble for not doing it, and indeed I learned the hard way, ending up in hospital several times for days on end with sepsis or allergic reactions. I just hadn't realised how quickly the most seemingly minor issue could escalate and become a much more serious problem.

On the first day they had given me a red card. Not for bad behaviour, but a red alert card for the twenty-four hour cancer treatment helpline. It's the opposite of what we are all used to when trying to make a GP appointment. The helpline is always manned, a medical person is always available, and you will be seen immediately.

After the first chemo it was not permitted to have anyone sitting with you for subsequent treatments. The ward is busy and has no room for extra people, although they can stay in the waiting room.

I could not believe how many people some patients brought with them. Some days I would arrive and there would be no seats, no space to sit down. I would think to myself, 'Gosh, it's busy today,' but no, apparently it was just a big family day out. It was always those families that were the loud ones – moaning, arguing, shouting, feet on the tables, eating strong smelling crisps very noisily with their mouths open and drinking fizzy juice then belching, completely oblivious to the fact some people were ill and needed quiet, or at the very least a seat as they waited for their treatment.

Occasionally a harassed receptionist would try to intervene and inform them that the seats were needed for patients to sit down. As you can imagine, this was not received well. I never understood why they were all there. Maybe I'm weird, but I didn't want anyone to come with me. I was far better left to get on with these things by myself. My loved ones didn't need to hang around the chemo unit, they saw enough of what it did to me at home. Let them go and escape for a while, even if it was just going to escape at work. In fact I found being by myself made me stronger. I got the train to hospital which was so convenient, no hassle with parking as the station was in the hospital grounds. Straight in and straight out. Sometimes as I walked through the grounds I became aware of other people arriving. It makes you realise just how many lives cancer affects. Everybody seems to know someone with it these days. A stark reminder that cancer has no prejudice. It's one of the few things in life that's free. Anyone can get it, and nobody wants it.

The hardest thing was seeing young people and children going through these aggressive but essential treatments. My heart broke for them and their families. I can't imagine how painful it must be to watch your child suffer. It makes me so thankful for my child's good health. Ironically, it was the children who always seemed to find something to be happy about. There was a young boy who I used to see at the unit, in his early teens probably, whose mother used to bring him. We would always acknowledge each other. I could see the deep lines etched on her face and the dark circles and bags around her eyes. Her whole persona exuded worry and pain. I wanted to reach out to her and hug her, I wanted her to have her joy back, the joy of having her child healthy again. Her son was always upbeat, making jokes, finding humour in the way he looked or at what was going on around him. He was brave and he brought a smile to your face. It made me think about how important it was to find my own sense of humour, how different that could make you feel. It's impossible to have bad thoughts when you are smiling.

Saints and Synners

THERE ARE SO MANY LOVELY people who give up their time to volunteer and do great work for cancer charities and cancer patients. During my time at the Beatson I was lucky enough to meet quite a few of them in different capacities. One lady in particular always managed to bring a smile to my face during my chemo. Her cheerful manner and the effort she put into her job was lovely to see. I am, of course, talking about a trolley dolly – one of a fabulous bunch of people who kindly bring you complimentary snacks and drinks during treatment, which is very much appreciated. I would always hear the trolley coming down the corridor as it had a squeaky wheel and dodgy steering. This was usually being wrestled with unsuccessfully by an elderly lady who I will call Agnes, for the purpose of identification.

Agnes had a very prominent limp and trying to push this stubborn cart was like manoeuvring a wonky supermarket trolley. It had a mind of its own. Laden down with hot water urns and sloshing milk jugs, in a busy ward, Agnes would persevere, arriving huffing and puffing at your side to greet you with a triumphant grin. It was actually Agnes that called herself a trolley dolly. Then she would have a fit of the giggles, before launching into an extensive list of the sandwich flavours on offer. She rarely had any of them left, but she felt each patient should have the full choice. Anything she didn't have she would try to get for you. This meant she would limp off back down the corridor dragging the disobedient cart with her, in an attempt to pick up more supplies from the kitchen. It was usually a fruitless excursion as supplies often ran out, and it was only what was on the trolley in the first place that was available. So back she would struggle, limping and squeaking, to tell you what you already knew... there's only cheese on white left. It was like watching Julie Walters in the Victoria Wood sketch *Two Soups*. It's not that I was laughing at her, I mean who was I to laugh at anyone as I sat there all bald and bloated, attached to tubes. I was just laughing at the ridiculousness of the situation. I had joined Slimming World to monitor my weight and stay in control of any weight gain, and there was no way I would let myself eat a 'syn' packed sandwich or a sugary custard, no matter how much I craved it. Agnes always tried to persuade me to have something from her dwindling supplies and I did feel guilty saying no thanks to her. It was as if she took it personally. However, the image of my Slimming World leader warning me, 'Be sure, your syns will find you out,' or 'Little pickers wear bigger knickers,' stopped me before I was tempted. Ah, the thought of that cool custard on my sore, blistered mouth was so tempting.

It took a while for me to realise that my priorities were all wrong. I had cancer for God's sake, who gave a rat's arse whether I ate an egg mayo sandwich or a Devon custard? Time for a reality check. I left Slimming World, became a synner, and started enjoying my visits from the squeaky trolley, much to the delight of a saint called Agnes.

FECkin Hell

ONE OF THE MOST ALARMING things after chemo was that my urine was bright red. When I first went for a wee I thought I had some strange internal bleeding, but apparently it is due to the colour of epirubicin. That is not the only freaky thing. It takes at least forty-eight hours, sometimes up to seven days, for your body to eliminate the waste products through urine, stools, vomit, semen and vaginal secretions. A leaflet is issued regarding "The safe handling and disposing of own body waste." As well as yourself, family members and carers should take careful precautions to avoid coming into contact with these waste products. Suddenly there are strict rules to follow:

- Wear disposable gloves.
- If waste products come into contact with skin or other body parts wash immediately with warm soapy water.
- Flush toilet twice with lid down and clean the bowl immediately whilst wearing gloves.
- "Double bagging" – sanitary waste should be placed in a plastic bag and tied tightly before placing in a second bag, tying tightly and disposing of in general household waste.
- Soiled clothing and sheets should be double bagged if not washed immediately.
- Condoms should be worn.

I started to form a picture in my mind of my family dressed like beekeepers in long gloves, decontamination suits and breathing equipment, hosing me down and scrubbing me with soapy water before letting me in the house. If I dripped on the toilet seat they'd have to buy a new seat. If I vomited, buy a new toilet. In fact, just throw out the furniture and move house, leaving me double bagged and ready for disposal.

Okay, perhaps a slight exaggeration, but it did make me wonder what was going into my body, and even worse what the hell was coming out. Whatever it was the side effects are not fun:

Feeling sick and becoming tired easily
Ah, just like being pregnant again.

Hair loss
Not a hair left on my body. Although, looking on the bright side, when it came to my legs, underarms and fandango I saved a fortune on waxing. However, losing my eyelashes and eyebrows was not pleasant. My eyes would get sore and red and my vision blurry. It was like having permanent conjunctivitis. No bonnie! Having no face or nasal hair might sound good, especially those stray long hairs that sprout white and wiry from your chin, or that grow down and hang out your nose, but let me tell you that a naked nose is a liability. It just runs all the time. Dreep Sammy Dreep. I was not even aware of it, I couldn't feel it running until it was too late and dripped onto my lap, repulsing anyone who happened to be looking. Nose hair has a purpose and I welcomed mine back with open nostrils when it grew in again.

Mouth ulcers and pain

I was given nystal mouth treatment and a revolting mouthwash. My tongue was cracked and painful. Nystatin is like thick mucus you drop in your mouth, swish round and swallow. Disgusting. My taste buds stopped working and anything I managed to eat or drink tasted of metal.

Nails

Some of my toenails looked like they had been shut in a door. They turned black. Not a good look in a summer sandal. Another weird thing was my toenails would come off whole! That was totally gross, they would literally just fall off. It wasn't painful and underneath would be skin that looked like a nail. Fortunately, it all pretty much returns to normal when you stop treatment and it's a real thrill when each bodily function or body part grows back or behaves as it should. As they say, you don't realise what you miss till it's gone. Unfortunately, some side effects are here to stay.

Chemo brain

Or cognitive dysfunction. This is when chemo affects the ability to concentrate and makes you more forgetful. Just like the brain shrinkage in pregnancy. I kid you not, all of a sudden your mind goes completely blank. You cannot find the word you want. You can't even remember what you were saying.

Hot flushes
Inner thermostat stuck on high.

Mood changes
It's Mama Moodswing and her Horror Moans. Sounds like my entry for the Eurovision Song Contest.

NIGHT SWEATS
It's goodbye oestrogen and all about 'the change', as overnight you are thrust into full blown symptoms of the menopause.

* * *

A *little ditty about feeling shitty*

Tick tock, tick tock, went my biological clock,
Then all of a sudden with no prior warning
Mother nature stopped conforming.
Everything's changing and it's outwith my power,
My clock went forward but not just by an hour.

Had PMS then PMT, been perimenopausal and I can't have HRT.
I'm high then I'm low and my memory's slow,
I'm teary, I'm weary, and this I'd like to query...
I'm too hot, I'm too cold, does it mean I'm getting old?

I just start to pee cos I can't hold in my wee,
I flush when I rush and my brain has turned to mush,
Hope it's not showing but I'm totally glowing,
From my feet to my head, I've turned bright red.

I go to bed completely dry
Then during the night I lie and fry.

I wake up looking like I've run a race,
My hair all stuck to my sweating face.

Steam rises from me, and I know it's not a dream,
The heat is even washing off my anti-ageing cream.
My duvet, sheets and pillows lie tangled in a heap,
What the hell happened when I was asleep?

I'm lying in a wet patch but it wasn't due to passion,
Cos the way I'm feeling now, sex is definitely on ration.
My knickers are wet and my fanny is dry
I've lost my sense of humour and I think I'm going to cry.

I have a shower and change the bed,
Put a cool gel pillow under my head.
I can only sleep three hours a night,
Always looking such a terrible sight.

I make strange noises when I have to bend down,
I've started farting as I walk around town.
My nerves are jangling and my hands are shaky,
I try to calm things down by getting reiki.

My face is bloated and I've swollen knees,
Mention the gym and I start to wheeze.
I'm on medication, I take tamoxifen,
I need to write it down so I remember when.

I drink too much wine then I start long rants,
I like to be comfy so I wear big pants.

Teaspoons attach to me like stickers,
Because there's magnets in my knickers.

I could ask Alexa what is wrong,
'I'm sorry, I cannot find that song.'
Guess I don't have to Google it to find the cause,
Hey girls – welcome to the menopause.

Brain Shrinkage

CHEMO CAN AFFECT THE ABILITY to concentrate and make you more forgetful. Yes, I do know I have already mentioned this. But when chemo brain and the menopause meet, the fallout really is alarming.

During my treatment I found that it was important to occupy my mind with other things. Throwing myself into work seemed a great idea. I had been an actress for twenty-five years and had not long moved into writing and performing. I had started my own company where the idea was to give very young children an educational but fun theatrical experience in the familiarity of their own environment. It was actually the head teacher at Molly's nursery who had persuaded me to do it. Molly had been asked what her parents did as a job, to which she replied, 'My daddy is a ballerina and my mummy is a prince,' obviously referring to the panto in which we met. This started a conversation about how young kids loved to see a show but taking groups of pre-school children to the theatre was both costly and a logistical nightmare. If only there were more professional companies who would come to them. So that's how it started. The great thing was that being self-employed meant I could schedule my shows to fit around my treatment. Some days were pretty crazy, driving to a venue and performing one or two shows before rushing off to provide more samples for phlebotomists, pathologists or pharmacists to analyse, then driving to another venue to do another show. As

Maureen used to say, 'They must be making black pudding in that place with all the blood they've taken.'

Just to get through some of those days gave me a huge feeling of accomplishment, but I was determined to enjoy them before the effect of the chemo wiped me out again. The other great thing about the job was that it involved interaction with very young children. Early years audiences are so refreshingly honest!

Each show was based on the Curriculum for Excellence and we covered topics such as good manners, oral health, and the importance of being kind to each other. There were only two of us involved – me and Alan – so we only performed when he was at home. We played all the characters, sourced costumes, props and set, yet the hardest thing was making it all fit into the back of our Hyundai i10. The car was so full that sometimes I would have to take the train! However, despite the unusual travel arrangements, working with the children was good fun and incredibly rewarding.

After I lost my hair I didn't want to alarm the children with my bald head and red shiny face, and thankfully each character I played wore a different wig, but as the kids loved to see what was behind the set at the end of the show I had to be careful. Often I was asked where the girl from the show had gone. I was more than happy to deny all knowledge of her, because another huge challenge was remembering lines due to my brain shrinkage. Some days Alan would look stunned at the nonsense I was coming out with. I just seemed to be making it up as I went along, desperately trying to remember words, songs or even worse, what was meant to happen next.

One day Alan came off stage during a quick change to find me dressed in completely the wrong costume. A fried egg instead of a pig in a blanket. My brain froze and it was complete panic as he had to run out front and start singing whilst I changed back as quickly as possible. It may all sound very trivial, but at a crucial part of the plot appearing as a fried egg would have confused everyone, including me. Have you ever experienced the wrath of a three year old heckler?

Poor Alan, working with me was becoming a liability and with the menopausal madness on the top he didn't stand a chance. No wonder he went away on tour so much. Thankfully people were very supportive and still continued to ask us to come back.

As each month passed I had a mini celebration in my head that another chemo cycle was over. However, another milestone was looming – my fiftieth birthday. I had been looking forward to turning fifty and had always thought of it as another coming of age, filled with exciting new opportunities. I was planning to rise again like a phoenix from the ashes.

Happy Birthday

On the first day of fifty the postman gave to me:
A bowel cancer testing kit.
On the fifth day of fifty the postman gave to me:
A pile of plans...
Plan your retirement,
Plan your funeral,
Plan your will,
And a bowel cancer testing kit.

IN THAT FIRST WEEK THE postman was never away from my door, stuffing my box, if you'll excuse the phrase, with ageist junk mail. I had become a senior citizen overnight. If you didn't already have a hang up about getting older, well you certainly would now.

So apart from the senior living advice and the menopause what did I actually get for my fiftieth? Well, let's just say some of the things were as useful as a partridge in a bloody pear tree. I got lots of birthday cards, again all decorated with pictures of flowers and butterflies or beautiful landscapes. Usually my mantelpiece would be adorned with wine o'clock messages, or 'Prosecco made me do it', but that year there was not a hint of humour or a rude message to be found. Most unsettling, and without trying to sound unappreciative, a couple of the gifts were a wee bitty strange too.

Scrabble-style fridge magnets with the letters F and C, which meant 'fuck cancer'?

Some cut out and keep postcards of merkins, offering a variety of styles?

Maureen's old boobs?

Yes, David thought they might come in handy if I needed a spare. Apart from the fact they were a different cup size, there was something not quite right about wearing my dead mother-in-law's prosthetic boobs. Possibly because I hadn't even had a mastectomy yet! You see everyone was at it, planning for the future.

It wasn't all doom and gloom by any means. I was incredibly spoiled and I was humbled by the kindness and thoughtfulness of others. One friend who had already been through breast cancer bought me a pot of bulbs with a card that read, 'When these bulbs flower so will you, because your treatment will be finished.' I thought that was lovely because it felt like a real and tangible time span to focus on. It made it seem not quite so far away.

On the subject of bulbs, probably the most generous thing that people did for me was to form and fund 'The Garden Gang'. This consisted of a group of our friends who decided to club together and renovate my garden. Some donated their time, some donated money and some bought plants. Hairdresser Tracey even took to social media, posing completely naked with packets of seeds covering her bits, Calendar Girls style, to ask for any donations of bulbs. Her customers responded so generously we could have started our own garden centre. The idea was that whilst I was recuperating I would be able to look out at a beautiful garden, instead of the overgrown jungle it had become, which would lift my spirits and make me feel good.

On the weekend they had chosen for the project it was the worst weather imaginable. However, that didn't stop them. They worked so hard, planting, chopping and clearing the overgrowth and best of all putting up a new fence, then they partied even harder. I was sent out of the way and told to put my feet up. They didn't want the mess and disturbance to stress me out. I felt so damn guilty sitting around while everyone worked that I busied myself making rounds of tea and coffee, even though they had brought all their food and drinks with them. My kitchen was the catering headquarters as bags of bacon rolls, hot soup and casseroles of ready-made hot food were unpacked. I was so grateful to them all. It was one of the best presents ever. Every night for several weeks the foxes dug up all the bulbs, but I just stuck them back in every morning. Not knowing what any of the bulbs were, or where they had originally been planted, not to mention which way up, it was a lovely surprise to see what was going to appear in bloom.

Alan and Molly also organised a wonderful surprise party in a private room of a local restaurant. I had no idea about it, and I hadn't planned to do anything as being mid-cycle of chemo and trying to keep working was pretty tiring. However, Alan and Molly were not going to be deterred. They had arranged a short two-hour drinks party and warned friends that it might have to be cancelled at short notice if I was ill. There was only one stipulation – wear a wig.

Some people were not sure if it was appropriate, and worried I might be offended, but they trusted Alan's judgement and entered into the spirit. It was the most fabulous gesture of solidarity and I felt so supported by the effort every single person in that room had made. It was packed as Alan had invited loads of people, not thinking they would all turn up. Friends and family had travelled from up north and down south to be there, despite it being for such a short time.

My big sister had wanted to fly over but unfortunately she would have had to be kept away from me for the first couple of days, just to make sure she hadn't picked up any germs on the flight, as my immunity was really low again. She only had a couple of days off work so she wouldn't have had time to spend any of it in quarantine! But that's my big sis for you, the only person I know who would fly over from Australia for a weekend. At my fortieth birthday, another amazing surprise party courtesy of Alan, my big sister jumped out of a giant box. I was overwhelmed – she had flown over from Oz for two days just to see me. All those weeks of top-secret negotiation between Jane and Alan and I knew nothing about it. Then, ten years later, he pulled it off again.

It was actually quite hard to recognise some people at the party, a sea of faces in a small space, looking like birds of paradise parading about with their exotic and colourful hair. The room was hot and crowded and I knew what they were going through. I could see people becoming more uncomfortable, beginning to rub at their heads and fiddle with their wigs, but just like etiquette at a wedding nobody dared remove their headwear until the bride's mother did. Or in this case, me.

So I dared to bare and put them all out of their misery, and with much relief a rainbow of acrylic hair was tossed into the air.

One final word of warning: please be careful when wearing a wig or prosthesis. Let the kids blow out the birthday cake candles!

Totally FEC-T

As each cycle of FEC was completed the oncology team seemed quite happy with the progress. My plum was measured at each appointment and the oncology doctors thought it was shrinking. When I say measured, there is no fancy machine to do this, a tape measure or school ruler does the job. Needless to say, there are probably a lot of guesstimates involved, but who cares if it's the news you want to hear. At one point they even thought a mastectomy might not be required. This was not a view shared by my consultant surgeon. She disagreed that there was any evidence of shrinkage, and in fact was not happy with the lack of progress. She even debated moving my surgery forward as she felt this particular chemo wasn't making enough difference. It was probably one of my first real low moments and another reminder of why I didn't get involved with the details. Any disappointments could be a cruel blow and they had a detrimental effect on my mental wellbeing. I didn't care if I was burying my head in the sand again, because I knew it was how I had to get through it.

Thankfully life outside the hospital was busy. Alan was travelling away a lot of the time with Scottish Opera work and Molly was dealing with the trials of starting a new school. On some days she would be really upset because nobody was being friendly and on other days she was very happy. My head was completely focused on her. If she was happy and having a good day then so was I. There were so many new experiences for her, including hockey matches on a Saturday morning, and her days were filled. When the inevitable bad side effects of chemo took their toll in the second week of a cycle, my friends and special shopping trips were a great distraction for her.

After three cycles of FEC the oncology team changed what they were giving me and added in Docetaxil. It did exactly what it said on the tin and left me totally fec-t. They also started me on steroids, which I had to take the day before chemo and for two days afterwards, supposedly to prevent an allergic reaction and reduce some of the side effects. The day after chemo a district nurse would call round and give me a bone marrow injection in the stomach. She performed this as if she was popping a balloon. Sadly my belly didn't deflate...

I'm not sure if it was the strength of this new dose of chemo, but I became ill again. So much of the treatment is trial and error, it's certainly not a case of one dose suits all. My oncology team were always quick to react and immediately reviewed my drugs, weakening the dosage. I was admitted to hospital again, which let's face it was becoming a regular occurrence. However, at least some of the time it was more of a precaution, and not just because one of those minor ailments I mentioned maybe wasn't so minor after all.

One of the worst things about this whole crazy ordeal was not being at home for Molly. The fear and guilt of not being there for my child made me angry. It was my job to look after and protect her, and suddenly she was having to take on a responsibility and a level of maturity way beyond her years. Feelings of guilt and helplessness, watching Alan juggling his working life with being a parent and a carer, whilst I lay in a hospital bed, tortured me.

During one of my hospital stays Alan had to go away to Hong Kong with the opera. The new chemo had blasted me, my hand had reacted to a faulty canula that had leaked, and my finger had turned poisonous. I was running a temperature, feeling dreadful, and there was no choice. I had to be admitted to hospital for six days and put on intravenous antibiotics and fluids. This meant leaving Molly. Like I said, we are blessed with a very supportive network of friends and family, but this was different. It was like sending her away to stay with someone. I was ever so grateful when once again Paul and Linda offered to help. They insisted they would look after her, despite having their own family trauma to contend with. Sadly, Paul's brother had been given a terminal diagnosis and had recently passed away. So there they were again in the same hospital, where they had brought him for chemo, visiting me, and seeing the same staff that had looked after him. No matter how grateful I was to them I was riddled with guilt for asking them to help. It must have been so hard for them with their emotions and grief so raw, but they were adamant. Molly was their niece, they loved her dearly, and she adored them. Yet I still felt I was failing Molly.

It's agony when your child is brought to visit you, when you can sense her neediness to be with you and then her reluctance to leave you. I could see that she was trying to be strong in front of me. It tears at your heart. At visiting times there were always too many other people around. Too many visitors who meant well but who didn't understand that was her time. My little girl was craving time alone with me. She wanted to get in the bed beside me and I wished I could pull the drips out of my arms so I could just hold her closely and shut the world out. When it was time for her to leave again the floodgates opened, and then it was me that had to be strong for her. Just a little girl who needed her mum.

Walking her out one day, I passed the nurses' station and caught sight of our reflection in the glass. My breath stuck in my throat and my blood ran cold. Was that really us? It was like watching a scene from a movie. Who was that bald, bloated person, clutching a distressed child? Was this really happening? I watched her being led away, her tear-stained little face looking back at me, and forced myself to smile and wave, trying to sound reassuring to prevent her lingering any longer.

As the doors to the ward swung shut I turned away with a stabbing pain in my solar plexus that felt as if an invisible umbilical cord was being ripped out of me. I looked at the nurses and saw that two of them were actually crying. However professional they are, they are still human and what they see must really get to them sometimes.

One of the nurses recognised Paul from when she nursed his brother. She was in my room and happened to ask how he was doing. When I told her that he had passed away, she actually broke down and then apologised for getting upset. I just gave her a hug. It must be so hard for them, I am not surprised if they get affected by their work, or if they feel attached to some of their patients. I certainly met some incredible people in hospital who left a lasting impression. Especially some of the ones who weren't going to make it. The courage they showed as they talked frankly about how long they had left was so surreal. Some of them didn't even look ill. One lady I met with terminal pancreatic cancer was so calm and matter of fact about it. Some days she would leave the hospital to have dinner at the hotel where her husband was staying, which was in the hospital grounds, before returning to the ward at bedtime. I remember the profound effect it had on me when she stopped her husband mid-sentence with a stark reminder that she would no longer be around by Christmas, so he was to stop including her in the arrangements.

Thankfully there were happier times too. I got quite close to one lady who used to watch my visits with Molly and always be there with kind words afterwards, telling me stories about her own family. She also had breast cancer but was having her treatment in a different order to me. She had a mastectomy first and was then getting chemo. But chemo weakens your bones, and she was going to be in hospital for weeks after she had fallen and broken her leg. She warned that something similar could happen to me, and sure enough it did about a year later, fortunately after I had finished treatment. I fell and broke my ankle whilst walking the dog on a flat grass football pitch... enough said!

I don't know why the pair of us found her situation so funny, but she looked hilarious with a bald head and a big stookie. The poor soul needed help with everything. She had stitches from her mastectomy which of course meant that she couldn't use crutches, so she was confined to a wheelchair that a nurse had to push. We were in a room on our own, just the two of us, and when she needed the toilet she would have to press her call bell then be helped into her chair and wheeled to the loo. Unfortunately the nurses were really busy and sometimes it could take a while to answer. We would start to giggle and the giggling would get more hysterical. Once I tried to help her and managed to get my drip stand tangled in her wheelchair, which of course set off the alarm on my machine. We were in trouble as patients are not allowed to help each other in case of accidents, although the only accidents we were involved in were of the bladder variety.

I remember a young nurse, a lovely chatty girl who we particularly liked. She had no filter, which amused us, and she just said whatever she was thinking. One morning as she stared at herself in the toilet mirror she was moaning about needing to get her highlights re-done, 'Check ma hair, it's a pure mess, I can't believe I had the brass neck to go out like this. What a pure riddy. Look at the state of me, coming to ma work looking like this.'

'Well, we're not going to judge you,' we sniggered, as we stared at each other sitting up in bed like a couple of potato heads, not a single hair between us.

She was mortified when she looked over at us and realised what she had said. Then, trying to recover herself, she exclaimed, 'At least you guys never have to worry about your roots, see the bloody cost of highlights... you're better off wi'oot hair!'

Perhaps a classic example of quit while you're ahead.

The Plastic Surgeon

A SCAN AND A SMEAR test had revealed dodgy goings on somewhere in my downstairs department, which would need further investigation. Hearing that news was a game changer for me. All of a sudden it was time to start taking back some control. Dealing with breast cancer was one thing but the suggestion of anything else was a step too far. I could not give head space to this new information – nothing was going to mess with my positive mental attitude. We were dealing with upstairs first, so until that was sorted, attending to my noo-noo was a definite no-no. It would have to wait its turn. Anyway, it would take some time to get an appointment after being referred to gynaecology, which meant I could keep my mind focused on the task in hand: new breasts.

First it was a meeting with my plastic surgeon to see if I had made any decisions. I was actually just pleased that I had remembered to return the DVD on time.

My options were having reconstructive surgery at the same time as mastectomy, usually preferable as it saved having two separate procedures, or to delay reconstruction until after all my treatment was finished.

However, when I found out that radiotherapy could damage the new breast, even shrink it, the decision was easy. There was no way I was going to go through reconstruction then risk my new breast being damaged, shrivelling up and falling off. Ok, perhaps that's a slight exaggeration, but I was only getting one shot so it had to work. I would delay reconstruction and wait till radiotherapy finished. Anyway, I had to choose which part of me I wanted to use. I always struggle to make decisions, and this was not an easy one to make.

Do you know they can make a boob out of your back? I misunderstood at first and wondered if that meant it would be facing the wrong way round... but no, apparently they just slice a bit of flesh, leave it attached, and swing it round. They don't waste any bits either, they'll use anything: bingo wings, thighs, stomach... now that's the one for me I thought, a tummy tuck at the same time!

I think it would be fair to say that my plastic surgeon had a definite way with words. His way. He pulled at my flesh like a potter throwing a piece of soggy clay onto his wheel, and said, 'Ah, I see you've had surgery there already,' indicating my two stomachs. I tried to suck in at least one of them.

'No!' I protested. Cheeky bugger. He had no idea how degrading the whole process was, being stripped to the waist and drawn on, then pulled and prodded and peered at by a bunch of male medical students (of course there's always an audience present), an entourage to stroke his ego.

'Ah, you mean it's all bought and paid for by yourself. I see there's plenty spare flesh on your back too. Well, we will certainly have plenty of choice.'

Don't hold back, why not go the whole hog and call me a fatty, lardy blubber back? A plastic surgeon eh? Well, he may not have been made out of plastic but he was certainly as damaging to the environment with his toxic outpourings. I mean he could have at least pretended, 'Oh Mrs McKenzie, you are very thin, we might have a hell of a job getting enough spare skin to make a boob.'

Can you believe he wasn't even going to pull my other one up either? I wanted breasts so pert my nipples would get stuck up my nostrils when I breathed in, but he was planning to match this new breast to my old one, a sock with a ping pong ball in the toe. I would look like a cow's udder after it's been milked. Not one but two of them slapping against my waist.

That was it, a decision delayed but very much made. Gathering up as much of my dignity as I could muster, I left.

Looking Good and Feeling Better

Nᴏᴠᴇᴍʙᴇʀ ᴛʜᴇ ᴛᴡᴇʟꜰᴛʜ 2015 ᴡᴀꜱ a momentous date in my diary. The day of my last chemo. Just one last round of steroids, bone marrow injections, sickness and feeling lousy.

Inevitably there was one more admission to hospital. The oncology team saw me getting wheeled down for a chest x-ray and said, 'You're not back again? At this rate we'll have to invite you to the staff Christmas party.' On the bright side, that was actually it. No more chemo. I had completed the first part of treatment.

Feeling re-energised and more positive I decided it was time to start making an effort with my appearance. Still being hairless I needed all the help I could get, so I signed up for the *Look Good Feel Better Workshop*.

One of the women I had met had highly recommended it and raved about the fabulous goodie bags of cosmetics you were given. Most of the items were no use to her but she was delighted anyway as she gave them away for Christmas presents.

The workshops are a superb idea. They are run by volunteers with a background in beauty, and some big cosmetic houses that are supporters of the charity donate products.

Arriving at Maggie's centre I was shown to a room and told to take a seat. In front of me on my table was a mirror, a twelve-step face chart for making notes and a white gift bag which was sealed. It's very exciting to open the bag and see what you have been given, as the contents of each are slightly different.

The beautician explained that the two-hour workshop would race by and that we may wish to make notes on our chart. To ensure that we all worked together at the same time, we were told to take our products out in the order we would use them, putting skincare on the left side of the mirror and the cosmetics on the right. Once a product had been used we were to place it back into our gift bag. Although we had been given perfume or body lotion too, we were asked not to open it in the class as some people would be sensitive to the fragrance.

Mixed reactions filtered along the row, from immense pleasure to disappointment, as the bags were emptied and contents examined. Realising that your neighbour got something better than you, while trying to disguise rather obvious feelings of product envy, we were like a bunch of children with a lucky dip.

'Lancôme cleanser, wow'

'Oh, mine's Avon. But I don't mind. I'm allergic to Lancôme eye makeup remover anyway.'

'What did you get?'

'No way, Estée Lauder mascara, lucky thing.'

'Me? Oh I got Boots No.7, but I quite like blue mascara anyway."

'What perfume did you get?'

'Oh, I've never heard of that one. I'll give that away.'

'I never wear blusher. Not with my hot sweats. Look at the colour of that, fuchsia.'

'I love that bronzer.'

'Lucky you, I'll swap if you want... fine then stick. It looks orange on your skin anyway.'

With all my products laid out in front of me, the volunteer beauticians started to take us through a skincare and makeup application routine.

'Now ladies, this is all about you. These products are for you. Don't be tempted to give them away to your daughter. It's time to spoil yourself and enjoy a bit of pampering. The first thing we are going to do is remove all our makeup with our cleansing, toning and moisturising routine. So if you just watch me, then copy what I am doing.'

At that point she pounced on some poor unsuspecting woman and covered her face with cream. I fought the temptation to turn to my neighbour and slap cleanser all over her, reckoning it was far too early in the proceedings for nonsense.

Like an air hostess demonstrating the safety procedures on an aircraft, our beautician held up cotton wool pads using hugely exaggerated sweeping motions across her face. Did you know there was a certain direction to sweep your cotton wool? She didn't say what would happen if you went the wrong way. You must use flowing, continuous movement to improve circulation and give a healthy glow. Apparently. There were even rules when it came to applying your moisturiser, tapping skin with fingertips only, never rubbing or dragging, not forgetting the neck and throat but avoiding the eyes (only eye cream was allowed on them!)

My skin is lucky if it gets a bit of three in one micellar water wiped across it. My makeup removal routine is rapid and not always very thorough, especially after a night out, thus the panda eyes and orange marks on my pillow in the morning. I don't spend time playing the piano on my face whilst using the heat of my finger tips to melt my moisturiser. However, staring at my turkey jowls and my stretched baggy eye skin in the mirror, I realised that's probably where I had been going wrong all those years.

Next was the concealer, foundation and powder stage. I usually don't use powder, I find it has an annoying habit of seeking out all the lines and crevices in my face and settling in them. All that fine dust seems to stick to the hairs that shouldn't be there. Maybe this was the ideal time to try again, with not a chin hair or a moustache in sight. But really, a magnified mirror? It just shows how deep the damage is. At two times magnification my fine lines become cracks and my face resembles an autumn leaf that's been dried out by the sun.

To avoid a shade malfunction or embarrassing tide mark (God forbid!) she demonstrated the importance of colour-matching foundation to skin tone. I didn't think they made products in flushed scarlet. I was told to apply a small amount of colour corrector to red patches, which in my case meant covering my face in green cream before applying my foundation, which was in palest ivory. I looked like a waxwork.

It wasn't an ideal match, but what's in your bag is the luck of the draw. The make-up would be set by face powder in 'rosy glow.' Presumably this would restore the colour I had just tried to blank out. Then it was time to apply the blusher. Mine was the brightest shade of pink I had ever seen. I looked like I had been punched.

Not to be deterred I carried on. It was eyeshadow next followed by eyeliner, which is always a challenge for me due to my shaky hands. When I try to draw lines on my eyes it looks like a five-year-old was in a hurry with their colouring-in. And with no eyelashes the eyeliner was inevitably severe, no matter how much I tried to soften it.

Finally my favourite section – the eyebrows. I have never ever used brow pencils. I always looked ridiculous with darker eyebrows, but this was a whole new ball game. We were actually going to have to create brows from scratch. We were shown how to measure from our nose to the inside edge of the eye and put a dot, followed by angling the pencil and making a second dot on the arch of the brow bone. A third dot was placed at the outer edge of the eye. Then you simply join the dots with feathery strokes to resemble fine hairs, and keep building colour and thickness to suit your needs. They even provided a useful tip: don't worry if both brows are not the same, as they are sisters not twins. Mine did not even look like distant relatives!

The mascara stage was obviously not relevant to me so it was onto the lipstick and lipliner. To compensate for what was happening at the top of my face I was rather hoping for a big bold red colour. Sadly 'nearly nude' and 'barely there' were not going to produce the statement lips I had hoped for.

With my green-white pallor and rouged cheeks, purple eyeshadow and squinty eyeliner, I had created a face that even Baby Jane Hudson would be ashamed of. As I looked in the mirror, I was trying to suppress an ill-timed fit of the giggles. The heat in the room was increasing and the chemo sweats were becoming more obvious. Not wanting a repeat of parents' night, I removed my wig. I looked like a hard-boiled egg that had been decorated for Easter.

However, I do have a lovely shaped head apparently, something I would never have known before all this happened. Every cloud and all that.

Some women followed suit removing their wigs, delighted to be more comfortable, but others preferred to keep their hair on (so to speak). Some had sensibly brought their turbans, and some still had a full head of real hair.

One lady I spoke to was scared of losing her hair and was trying to prepare herself for the trauma of hair loss in the near future. She didn't know how to tell her twelve-year-old son about her cancer. She was terrified about what it would do to him as she was a single parent. My heart went out to her and I explained that I had been completely honest with my eleven-year-old, and spoke about Molly's reaction to it. We talked about involving his school for support and how staff can monitor his behaviour, and also about other help and support that's available for him. By the end of the workshop, after hearing other peoples' stories, she felt ready to go home and talk to him.

Sitting next to me were two ladies who turned out to be mother and daughter. They had both been diagnosed with ovarian cancer. The mother was only a few years older than me and the daughter was twenty-six with two young children under five. They just wanted to be there to support each other and look their best.

It was a room full of people whose lives were tinged with sadness, yet there was still so much positivity and laughter present. Our confidence was boosted and illness was forgotten. For those two hours we weren't just patients, we were women again, enjoying things that normal women do. We were all different, we were all riddled with insecurities, yet we shared one common bond. We were looking good and feeling better.

Swiss Cheese

HAVING COMPLETED CHEMO FOR MY top half, it was time to have a look downstairs and see what was happening with my under-carriage. I was booked in for my gynaecology scan at the end of November. This was actually a blessing as I was crazy busy with work and it left me no time to worry about what they might find. It was just another waiting game for results.

We were performing two shows a day, sometimes three, due to the fact that all our December bookings had to be completed before the seventh, as that was the date I was due to have a mas-tectomy. All the venues had been very helpful about us changing dates, which was a huge relief as I hadn't wanted to let anyone down by having to cancel. Although, as people pointed out, I did have a valid reason and wasn't exactly pulling a sickie. I was able to immerse myself in the childrens' pre-Christmas excitement and take time out from reality. I am sure that is what got us through those difficult days.

At my last meeting with the surgeon before my operation, she discussed the fact that she had been hoping for an eleventh hour reprieve to avoid a full mastectomy, but that wasn't a possibility. Unfortunately, she would have to perform a full mastectomy and lymph gland removal on my right side. By this point I didn't care what they had to do, just as long as it was successful.

After finishing our final shows on the sixth of December I fasted from midnight and was admitted for surgery at half past seven in the morning. I was hoping for an early surgery slot as my nerves were starting to take hold. I was incredibly thirsty and craving a shot of caffeine. Eventually I was called from the waiting room into what I can only describe as the wardrobe department, where they issue you with your costume. I was then put on a trolley and tucked up, which felt extremely strange, before being pushed through to join other patients lying on trolleys, all waiting to be collected by the surgical team. Although we were all in for different operations we were all dressed in the same glamorous way: white surgical stockings, disposable gowns and shower caps. It felt like that awful moment at school when you are waiting to see which team will pick you – all the popular ones are chosen first and you nervously wait, praying not to be left till last. As I lay there I watched the medical team in their scrubs and clogs putting on paper clothes and a school dinner lady hat, half expecting one of them to come out with, 'D'ye want beans with that?'

To complete the look I had been decorated with some rather unsubtle purple graffiti. 'RHS' and big arrows that pointed to my breast and arm had been drawn in marker pen, indicating which side to operate on and what was to be removed. Better safe than sorry I guess but it freaked me out, it made it all a bit real. Then before I could think about running away a cannula was inserted and I was wheeled through.

I will always remember the powerful image of the journalist Victoria Derbyshire holding a sign that read, 'Hi, this morning I had breast cancer. This evening I don't.' Now it was my turn... I could say that. My breast was gone along with sixteen lymph glands. I don't know if that is a little or a lot, and I don't care. I don't need to know.

For the first time in months I was free of cancer and ready to start radiotherapy as soon as my scar healed. My surgeon described the breast she removed as a lump of Swiss cheese. The holes in the tumour had been made by the chemotherapy, but it hadn't destroyed it completely. She had made the right choice to remove the entire breast and surrounding lymph glands.

Molly and Alan came to visit me that night. I was groggy but deliriously happy. They dressed me up with a bed pan on my head and a scarf and took ridiculous photos. Maybe not normal visitor behaviour, but they were having fun with Fester. Molly found me especially amusing and took videos of me as the nurse helped me to the toilet. I had drains and drips to contend with and I felt off my face. The drainage bags were in a pouch with a shoulder strap which I kept forgetting about, only to be reminded when it fell off the bed, yanking at the drains and pulling at my new stitches. Just as well I was still numb as that happened frequently for the first few days.

The nurse expertly gathered up the tangle of tubes that I was wired to, like an attentive bridesmaid holding a train. Slowly I got out of bed and shuffled unsteadily towards the toilet. Still feeling the after effects of sedation I had difficulty walking and coordinating properly. I heard the sniggering behind me, but I was totally oblivious to the fact that my gown was open and my extra-large see-through white disposable pants were on display. Bridget Jones eat your heart out.

The three of us were laughing again and it felt good.

The White Swan

BEFORE THIS ALL HAPPENED, I was once told that I had a young womb. Now, I don't know how you go about ageing a womb, but I was happy to take the compliment. I replied, 'Thank you very much,' but judging from the reprimanding look and the raised eyebrow, I'm not sure my response was required. Since then I've always felt secretly a little bit smug.

However, that was nothing compared to how I felt on the twenty-third of December when I got the results I had been waiting for. My latest gynaecology scan had revealed nothing suspicious. Doctors were completely baffled by comparing the two sets of scan pictures and results. Where was the shadow or the mass or whatever they had seen previously? How could it all be clear? Perhaps the chemo had blasted it all away, or maybe the alternative healing had helped – the combination of reiki and a positive mental attitude. Quite frankly it didn't matter. We had the results we had dreamed about. My young womb was considerably older, but we were so grateful.

During chemo I was lucky to have been given regular reiki and relaxation treatments by my special friend and inspiring teacher, Margaret Craig. I looked forward to her sessions and benefited greatly from receiving such beautiful healing energy. It made me feel safe, protected and free, as I would be transported to a place of great beauty and peace. If you have never tried it I cannot recommend it highly enough. I am so deeply grateful to her for all the time she spent with me, and for some beautiful meditations that took me far away from pain and suffering, and that replaced my fear with hope and positivity.

One of my favourite meditations during a reiki treatment was being taken to a beautiful lake surrounded by mountains and vivid colours. A boat would be waiting to take me into the centre of the lake where I would just lie and rest. No noise, perfect peace, just floating there with only the soft lapping sounds of the water and the sun on my face, I would drift off to sleep. Except instead of a boat it was always a huge white swan that came to collect me. When the swan appeared I would curl up on its soft back, its white feathers warm and comforting, and it would fold these enormous protective white wings around me. I felt like Thumbelina curled up in a flower. Then the swan would swim slowly and gently around this magical lake. I have never felt more safe and secure. When it was time to leave, it would take me back to the shore, relaxed and rested and peaceful.

I know this kind of thing is not for everyone, but it worked for me.

My Shark Bite

THE RECOVERY PROCESS AFTER MY mastectomy was hard work. Well, nobody said it was going to be easy. Persevering with the uncomfortable daily exercises was tough, and progress felt so slow. Some days I had to really push myself to do them, and I felt quite soul-destroyed by the lack of movement. Just to be able to raise my arm above my head was going to take a lot of effort and practice. During the first few weeks I began to wonder if I would ever get full movement back. The pain and strange pulling sensations in my chest and arm felt like a rope being stretched. This, combined with a complete lack of feeling in my armpit, shoulder blade and side, meant that I was permanently uncomfortable and feeling pretty low.

The first time I dared to look in the mirror was awful. It was difficult to accept what I was seeing. I think I was in shock. I knew what to expect having seen Maureen with her double mastectomy on numerous occasions. However, if I'm brutally honest it used to freak me out. I always pretended to her that it didn't bother me but deep down I struggled with it.

Now it was me. I can't lie, I felt a complete freak. One boob just looked weird. I could only take short glimpses before I hid my chest away again. Sometimes I would even forget that I looked different, then I would suddenly catch my reflection in the bathroom mirror... so I tried not to look.

When you lose something like a body part you become aware

of everybody else having it. Everywhere I looked there seemed
to be pictures of beautiful women with boobs. Glamour models,
Hollywood stars, celebrities. Everybody had perfect boobs. It
defined you as a woman. The thought of being attractive without
them was impossible to grasp. How could I ever feel attractive
with one boob?

My husband was amazing in how he dealt with it all. He made
me think about things in a different way. He said that when he
saw my chest it made him feel grateful, happy that the cancer had
been cut out. It was a reminder that it was gone. This made a
huge difference to me and slowly I started being able to look.

I referred to the scar as my shark bite. By not connecting the
scar to cancer I found it easier to accept. God knows why I chose
to think of it like that. I mean, if I had been attacked and mutilated
by a shark then I guess the psychological scars would run pretty
deep. But I wasn't about to start arguing with myself – it was a
trauma to the body and it didn't matter how I processed it, as long
as I accepted it.

I still struggle some days. A silly thing like passing a lingerie
department or bikini shopping for a summer holiday can be
a harsh reminder that I can't just wear what I want, I need to
choose carefully.

Let's face it, who wants to have to use specialist companies for
bras or swimwear? Sometimes it's just fun to pop into Primark
and pick up three bikinis, three pairs of flip flops, three sarongs,
a sunhat, glasses, and a beach bag, all for twenty-five pounds. It's
only when I get them home and find there's no prosthesis pocket
that I realise I can't wear it. I now usually wear a bikini top with
plenty of frills, which saves popping in a knocker. Mind you, I
have more need to worry about having two stomachs than two

boobs. It will still be a while before I'm ready to indulge in a spa day or massage.

You're probably wondering why I don't just get the reconstruction surgery and stop whinging! The simple answer is because I've had enough of surgery and being a patient, and so have my family. I want to participate in life, not just be a spectator, and there's so much living to catch up on. I suppose if I'm really honest, I am also concerned that if I do something for vanity reasons and something went wrong, I'd blame myself. There you go, that's the menopausal fear creeping in.

I need to just be grateful that I'm well and have a wonderful supportive husband who claims that he was always more of a leg man anyway! When I win the lottery I will take time off and get my boobs and bunions sorted. In fact, I'll give my entire body-work a bloody good overhaul. Maybe I will travel to America and get fixed by those two doctors, Dr Terry Dubrow and Dr Paul Nassif from the programme *Botched*. Until then, I am happy to just be me.

Knitted Knockers

It's incredible what you hear about from the person in the next hospital bed. My roommate with the stookie was a constant revelation. The most interesting thing she told me about was her knockers – they're knitted. That was it, I nearly fell out of bed laughing. Knitted knockers! I thought she was definitely winding me up, but she told me to Google them as soon as I got home and I am so glad that I did.

The company has teams of volunteer knitters, and they forward your order to knitters within your area. These people are amazingly talented and custom knit each knocker to your individual requirement. They are then beautifully packaged in a gift bag, with a personal note from your knitter, and a printed message that reads, 'Each knocker is made with love and filled with hope.' I will never cease to be amazed by what people can knit. They come in a range of colours too: light, bright, pastel, black, dark, striped, available with or without nipples!

My friend Petra very kindly decided to knit me some, so I didn't have to order them. God knows what her children thought. 'Holly, run to the wool shop and get some more wool, I am just knitting your Aunty Gilly some knockers.' She downloaded the pattern but the end result was more 38GG than 38B. It must have been a stuffing issue. Jeez, the nipple itself was like a lethal weapon. One wrong move it would have taken your eye out.

Let's just say they would make lovely soft scatter cushions for the spare bedroom, an interesting talking point for your guests over breakfast the next morning. Maggie the dog likes sleeping on them. I sometimes find them in her toy box. Petra persevered and the next set were a big improvement; I wore them out on their maiden voyage, whilst shopping, one warm Saturday afternoon. Half way round Marks and Spencer I nearly passed out from overheating!

Petra had stuffed them with fur-lined thermal tights and it was like wearing a sauna suit, or an extra couple of jumpers under your coat. Handy in the winter perhaps. In the end I went back to the website and had them made in the proper size.

I am now the proud owner of some real beauties, it's like the chest I never had. Just as well I've got a partner... can you imagine getting carried away with your new date and them coming across those knitted beauties!

I honestly cannot recommend knitted knockers highly enough. They are so soft and light to wear, because what nobody tells you is that it's bloody sore on your scar to wear a bra with a heavy prosthesis. Specialist companies, which always have double-barrel Christian names like *Nicola Jane*, send you brochures of eye-wateringly expensive or very unfashionable swimwear, lingerie and prosthetic breast options. As far as I'm concerned you can't beat an Asda post-surgery bra and a woolly boob. I believe you can get your national health prosthesis replaced every two years, but if it's used constantly, it's in a pretty saggy and baggy state by then. Mind you, at least that matches it up better with my real one.

Not only do they make knitted knockers, they also make aqua knockers for swimming. These are multi-purpose because they stuff them with shower scrunchies. So after your swim you can take your wee knocker into the shower, remove the scrunchie and you've got an instant loofah.

I cannot stress enough how important it is to buy a proper bra with pockets. I thought I would save money by wearing a normal bra. I popped my wee woolly knocker in and off I went. Very comfortable, so far so good, I forgot all about it.

However, unless you keep them restrained they can have a tendency to migrate. They will suddenly make a break for freedom... settling under your arm then falling out the bottom of your top when you stand up. I used to wonder why they had a little tail attached, but I think you're meant to secure them, tie them down like boats in a harbour. One night I was in a busy bar and after a couple of Cavas, feeling very relaxed, chatting away, the next thing... there it was, my ship had sailed, broken its moorings, and launched itself out of my top. I don't mean subtly, mine had worked its way out and was dangling there, restrained only by its woolly tail which had tangled round my bra strap. Try explaining your way out of that one. I couldn't exactly pretend it was my earring that had fallen out. My top was flattened against me on the side where the knocker had previously been. Suffice to say a pink and white striped knitted knocker with a large nipple attracted many curious stares from the busy bar.

A Curry, a Cava and a Concert

JUST A COUPLE OF WEEKS after my surgery it was Christmas. Of course that means one thing in our house: the dads arrive. We could have done without house guests and all the extra work, but it was Christmas and no one should be on their own unless they want to be. Given what we had all been through in 2015 it was right to all be together anyway. Cooking was definitely not going to be an option, so we decided to book a restaurant for Christmas dinner. We had never gone out at Christmas before, and wanting a change from traditional festive food we opted instead for a Christmas curry. Our friends Tracey and Ewan and his family also decided to join us. For some ridiculous reason we decided to wear Christmas jumpers. Feeling the heat as I do, I have no idea why I thought that was a good idea.

Alan and Molly had bought me a bright red wig for Christmas, which although stunning unfortunately did not suit me at all and clashed violently with my round red face and festive jumper. When I got hot I looked like a big red shiny bauble. I can't believe my family let me go out like that, and the worst thing was that I wasn't trying to be funny. The rest of the party were dressed more appropriately, although Tracey still opted for a pink wig, and Ewan turned up dressed as an elf.

In a restaurant where the waiters wear kilts and serve haggis pakora, where Santa had a turban peeking out from under his hood, and where an optional menu offered a curry, a cava, and a concert, it should not have been our table that was the subject of so many photographs. Apparently the 'concert' just meant a pre-theatre menu. I probably should also mention that Ewan is a part time magician and had brought along a couple of tricks. A wallet that burst into flames attracted a lot of attention, especially from the concerned staff as they brought us our bill. Next Christmas I'll order the curry and the cava as a carry out.

As January 2016 arrived, I felt ready and eager to start the radiotherapy. All of a sudden there seemed to be light at the end of the tunnel, which filled me with new positivity and strength. I was nearing the end of treatment.

Alan decided to organise something special before I started the final phase. He noticed that Olivia Newton John was playing at the Glasgow concert hall, as part of the Celtic Connections folk festival, along with Beth Neilson Chapman and Amy Sky. I knew nothing about the concert, so it was a total surprise, in more ways than one. When we got there we thought *Liv On* was something to do with Olivia's name. It was actually the title of a new album they had brought out, described as, 'To aid and comfort those experiencing grief and loss while using the power of music to heal.'

I had actually forgotten that Olivia had been through breast cancer until I saw her being interviewed after Kylie had been diagnosed. All three women on stage had been affected by cancer and lost loved ones to it. They were 'sisters in survival.' However, I hadn't expected all the songs to be about cancer and death!

As one reviewer wrote at the time, 'Grief is the word.'

I don't want to make the concert sound awful because it was absolutely brilliant. Those songs were so moving, I was an emotional wreck. A few songs in from the beginning, someone behind me kindly bent forward and passed me a tissue. Embarrassing, but they were very nice about it. I just hadn't been prepared for such powerful lyrics and emotional performances. If you haven't heard the album I suggest you listen to it, but for God's sake be warned, have a large gin and a box of tissues at the ready.

Alan had hoped to get a signed photo of Olivia for me, with a message from her to encourage me to stay strong, however he knew he wouldn't be able to get in contact with her. He'd even thought about leaving a note at the stage door, which he didn't, but it was a kind thought anyway. Towards the end of the concert, Olivia said, 'We told you our stories, so now let's hear some of yours.' The house lights went up and a microphone was passed amongst the audience.

I looked at Alan and said, 'Don't you dare!'

A couple of people stood up before him, but he was determined, and somehow the third and final person was him. As the mic was passed along the row, I cringed. Please don't draw attention to us... too late, as he burst into the first few lines of, 'I love you, I honestly love you,' directing it to Olivia (which actually turned out to be her next song), the concert hall burst into applause and cheered loudly.

'What a voice!' exclaimed Olivia, whilst Beth and Amy whooped in agreement.

Someone else shouted, 'He should be on that stage.'

I have to admit, he sounded amazing. Great mic, great acoustics, great voice. Then Alan proceeded to quickly tell them about the loss of our mums and my diagnosis. All three women listened to his story then Olivia came forward. She waved and said, 'Hi Molly.' Aagh! What a thrill, Sandy from Grease just said hi! Then to my surprise she said, 'This is for your wife. Hi Gilly, I just want to say that I am twenty-five years on from breast cancer, so keep on,' then she blew me a kiss.

I can't tell you how special getting that message felt. It was a heart stopping moment when she spoke to me. I felt inspired.

Ring the Bell

IN PREPARATION FOR RADIOTHERAPY I had my first planning scan, where I was tattooed with little dots that are permanent and look like blackheads. Very frustrating when I found myself trying to squeeze them. I lay on a table as machines were pulled around me and I was positioned and measured and repositioned, then drawn on again to make sure they were hitting the right bits with their beams. It was all very technical. This was followed two weeks later by a pre-treatment image check before starting radiotherapy the next day.

I was to have sixteen sessions of treatment, Monday to Friday for just over three weeks. Radiotherapy did not interfere with everyday life in the same way that chemo had, and apart from tiredness and a little tenderness that felt similar to sunburn, I had no ill effects at the time. It would be months before I felt nerve pain and strange cramps or tightening under my arm and chest. I also have a darker rectangle of skin where I got the radio, but all these side effects are apparently to be expected. It's funny when you are told something is perfectly normal or to be expected, it makes it easier to tolerate. You just accept it.

The staff were always so friendly and I very quickly felt a familiar bond with them. As soon as I arrived and removed my clothing, ready to be positioned for the machine, they put me at ease by talking about family, social lives, food and drink, all far removed from the reality of the situation. It always struck me that they had incredible memories. They must see countless patients yet they would still remember little details from previous conversations, even the date of my wedding anniversary. I was always treated like an individual and not a CHI number. The only unpleasant feeling was created by myself, in my mind.

Bizarre fears entered my head when the machine was positioned over me and the square of light pinpointed its target. I would hear the mechanical noises and the whirring sounds as it started but I never saw what the machine was doing as I always closed my eyes. I was terrified a stray beam could zap me and blind me. Sometimes I would panic that the machine would crush me or burn through my skin. My imagination would go into overdrive and I was always hugely relieved to hear the friendly voices as they came to reposition me before the next blast. Within no time the treatment session was over and there would be more cheery chat as I got dressed and prepared to leave. It was a surreal experience. I often found myself thinking, 'Did that just happen? Did I just get radiotherapy?' as the staff were telling me about what they were going to feed the cat that night or what they were planning to watch on tv... just normal people doing normal things.

It was so different from my experience in the chemo ward. In the waiting room boxes of chocolates and magazines adorned the tables, and you recognised and acknowledged fellow patients. No moaning and groaning about waiting times there. I would see the same faces every day, until it was their turn to pick up the large hand bell and ring it in celebratory style, signifying the end of their treatment, which was greeted with a round of applause. The next day there would be new faces to fit the empty spaces, and soon they would become familiar too.

On the sixteenth of February 2016 it was my turn to ring the bell ... but I didn't actually bother. I was the only patient left in the room as everyone else had finished treatment and gone home for the day. But I didn't need to ring a bell, there were trumpet fanfares, fireworks and champagne corks popping inside my head. Ironically it was also Maureen's birthday.

That was it, there was no more. I had finished treatment.

Moving Forward

As I LEFT THE RADIOTHERAPY department and walked down the nearly deserted corridors, I have to admit I felt very strange. Almost anti-climactic, mixed with a little bit of fear. What now? Having spent the previous year being told what to do by doctors, following rules and schedules of medication, attending appointments and having a daily routine and structure, it would all suddenly stop. It's almost too much to take in. Like a prisoner being released from prison, sudden freedom can be quite daunting. I was back in charge, back calling the shots, I didn't have to report to a hospital again. It's strangely intimidating. You don't realise how institutionalised you have become.

To prepare me for this next stage I was asked to attend a short meeting, organised by Breast Cancer Care, where they provided me with an information pack and advice about 'moving forward after breast cancer'. The folder is full of useful information and services to help you with both the physical and emotional side of your recovery after the hospital treatment has finished. I was informed that it was quite normal to want to come back and talk, that I might feel isolated after finishing treatment. This meeting was to reassure me that I was not alone and I could talk to professionals or to someone who had been through the same experience. Quite frankly, the idea horrified me. I mean Maggie's is a fantastic place, but I didn't want to go back thank you. It was full of folk with cancer. For the time being I had listened to enough cancer stories. Strange as this may sound, cancer is a bit like pregnancy. The news tends to spark off everyone else's reminiscences of their own experience. Of course, in the same way that every pregnancy is different, every experience of cancer is different.

I don't know what was worse: meeting up for coffee, cake and a bit of chat with the new mums or the cancer chums. Personally, I would try to avoid both.

'OMG, gas and air, really? I had absolutely no pain relief.'

'I followed my birth plan and breathed and floated.'

'She had an epidural, that's not really giving birth is it?'

'A caesarean definitely doesn't count.'

'Oh mine was easy, three pushes and she was out, not a stitch. Just a little scratch from her fingernail.'

'No stitches? That's nothing to brag about. That's just her past catching up with her.'

'I was in labour for seventy-seven hours, my baby was twelve pounds, I had to get forty-four stitches, and now I poo out my front bottom.'

You can find that same hint of competitiveness from the cancer chums, as each relives their experience. The suggestion of getting off lightly if you didn't have chemo, the question of how many radiotherapy sessions you needed. As comparisons were made there was an air of superiority if you suffered more. Lumpectomy versus mastectomy versus double mastectomy. Did you lose your hair, did you go completely bald, has it grown back in? Were your lymph glands removed, did you have a reconstruction, primaries, secondaries... aargh, stop! Please!

It's gone, it's over, that's all that matters.

Then there was the member of staff who told me, 'We can never say you are all clear. Anyone who tells you that is not correct. It really bothers me when I hear people saying they got the all clear, it's simply not true. We can't give you that guarantee.'

Can you believe that? Who in their right mind would say that to a patient who has just finished treatment? Obviously they had never had cancer. They didn't understand how important it was to hear the magic words. I decided that I would say it to myself instead, because I wanted and needed to hear those words.

So I didn't go back. I went forward. I coped, I realised what was important, and how precious good health was. I didn't talk about cancer, I blocked it out as if it had never happened. It was gone, and that's all that mattered.

Chemo Curls

AFTER THE TREATMENT WAS OVER, I couldn't help thinking about my hair and whether it would ever grow back in. I am delighted to say it did. Mind you, there were quite a few unfortunate stages and some looks were kinder than others. I was so excited by the first bit of fuzz reappearing that I didn't care that I looked like a newly hatched chick. I wanted to cast off my wig immediately, but as Alan and Molly pointed out, it was perhaps better to stick with it for just a little bit longer.

I had been warned about chemo curls, and the only way to describe them is, well... they're bizarre. I always had poker straight hair and had never managed to get even as much as a kink in it before. Now little ripples and waves were appearing on my very short covering of fuzz. It wasn't long before the fuzz grew and the ripples turned into curls, then into really tight curls, and eventually into a granny perm. That was not a great look, although I am lucky it didn't grow in grey like it does for some. My hair eventually grew back a dark blonde colour but being so short it just looked dark. It would be another year before it would accept colour. I longed for that little summer lift, a bit of bleach in the highlights. In fact, one day I was walking Maggie, and a man came up to me and said, 'Hey missus, you've goat the same hair as yer dug!'

He was right, but I didn't tell him why.

Another time, when we were on holiday, we would pass the

same couple each night on our way out for dinner. They had always seen me in a peroxide bob. However, one day at the pool they must have recognised Alan and Molly, but not me at first. When they did the wife hurried over and sat down uninvited on my lounger, exclaiming, 'Oh, have you been poorly?'

Obviously I was not wearing my wig. She then proceeded to tell us all about her own cancer experience. Just what you want to hear whilst sunbathing at the pool!

The next stage I went through was my Princess Diana phase, which I quite liked in an old-fashioned, retro sort of way. Sadly this eventually morphed into a Camilla, which I was not so keen on. As my hair grew longer my tight chemo curls grew down until eventually they became little knots at the ends of my hair, making it impossible for a brush to go through. There was no option but to get my hair trimmed. That really felt like a momentous day. Tracey had opened her new salon by that time and I was so excited to at last be a customer. She very carefully snipped at the ends of my precious new hair, knowing I was terrified to take too much off in case it didn't regrow. I needn't have worried. My hair grew and grew and it has now passed my shoulders and become a lot thicker and heavier. I have the odd curl and a lot more body in my hair than I did before. Apart from sometimes being a bit woolly, it is almost better than my hair was before chemo.

I credit a lot of my successful hair regrowth to my friend Richard, who constantly provided me with the most calming and relaxing Indian head massages, before, during and after my treatment. The massage increases oxygen and nourishment to the scalp and hair follicles, which in turn stimulates hair growth. It definitely worked for me and I really am a very lucky girl.

The Gift

WHEN I STARTED WRITING THIS it was hard, because I didn't want to remember. I was scared to revisit that place in my mind, scared it might bring the cancer back. I didn't know what I was going to find locked away in my memory. It was a bit like the feeling of pulling a stuck dressing off a wound and bursting open the stitches. But I'm glad I faced up to my fears, by confronting them I removed the power they had over me.

Now it feels like I am talking about someone else, and I suppose in a way I am. After being on this cancer journey I will never be the same. Life moves on, scars start to heal, memories become hazier and my recall of treatment becomes slightly rosier. However, one thing will never change, and that is my feeling of gratitude. Someone once asked me how I could possibly describe myself as lucky if I'd had cancer. I found this totally astonishing. I am here, I survived. I would call that lucky.

When I was in my late twenties and going through a bit of a rough time, my best friend's mum told me, 'Within every problem there is a gift for you.'

I didn't appreciate what she meant, replying flippantly, 'So where's my fucking present then?'

Well, all these years later Myra Collins, I finally found it... the gift of good health, the gift of life. And I am so grateful for it.

The Journey
By Molly McKenzie

LAST YEAR WAS A TOUGH year. Last year everything was happening at once. I was in hospital after my tonsil operation. I'd been kept in for a few more days because I'd had a bleed. I was hyper after all the painkillers and drugs I was on. I was on repeat and kept falling asleep every five minutes and then waking up questioning where I was.

Anyway, one morning I woke up to a doctor in my face. I got a fright and jumped back. I took a deep sniff through my nose... ugh! Three days without a shower, the adrenaline of an operation and stuck in a hospital bed... *I smelled amazing!* Not! The doctor examined my throat. I felt all clogged up and disgusting. He took a few notes and then later told me I was free to go. Mum started to panic as she had an appointment at the Western. She managed to phone my dad's cousins to come and pick me up from the Western but they live all the way out in East Kilbride so it took a while for them to arrive.

When Mum and I arrived at the Western I thought it looked kind of run-down. We sat in the waiting room, it smelled like paint. I looked around the room and everyone looked rather depressed and glum, mind you I was *extremely* happy and I kept seeing smiley faces everywhere.

Mum got called through and although she got up and pretended like nothing was wrong I knew something was up. I sat at reception and stared at the clock, I'm a little embarrassed to say but it took me ten minutes to realise the clock was broken. Reception was empty, not even a receptionist to gab at. I slumped down in my chair and sighed. Twenty minutes passed... nothing. Another ten minutes went by. Finally, after forty minutes, Dad's cousins arrived and I have never been so relieved to see them. They took me home and got me cosied up on the couch and forced the worst tasting medicine down me. It's so rank I can't even explain it. It didn't have a flavour, it was just bitter. Bitter, fizzy and it caught at the back of my throat.

Hours passed and Mum was still not back. I started to worry. When Mum was finally back I was thrilled to see her! I threw my arms around her but it was really strange as she was kind of awkward with me and normally she is so embarrassing and gushing with affection. I sat on the stairs and heard some swear words, 'Dad', 'Aberdeen' and 'telling her tomorrow'. I couldn't put two and two together, I didn't understand.

That night Mum was teary and touchy and Dad was angry and uptight. I just thought I was being needy because I had just come out of hospital. I felt like a pain and went to bed rather upset and vulnerable.

The next morning I woke up happier. I was having a good day. I had just skipped upstairs and was about to start makeup and hair, when Mum and Dad called me downstairs and all I was thinking was, 'You had to wait until I'd just settled down up here!'

Anyway, I doddled downstairs and Mum and Dad sat me down. Why were they being so serious and formal? Mum began to stutter... what was happening? Mum was an actress, a confident speaker, she never stuttered! She looked like she was going to burst into tears. Dad finished for her.

'Well, eh... Mummy has been diagnosed with breast cancer. It's in most of her lymph glands under her arm as well.'

I dived on top of both of them. I had never heard worse news in my life! (Not over-exaggerating.)

Dad continued, 'She is going to the Beatson and getting chemotherapy. Her hair is going to fall out, her eyelashes and her eyebrows too. She will then go in for her operation and then finish off with radiotherapy. Treatment is going to last about a year and it's going to be tough, but we will defeat it as a threesome!'

It was all too much. Not only was I going to be starting a new school in a couple of weeks but both my grannies died from breast cancer. It was very traumatic. Not only was I trying to fit in and make friends but I had seen my mum go from beautiful long, blonde hair to it coming out in my hand and then not a single hair on her head, which made her look like a shiny egg. But we found a positive, optimistic and funny side even while she was lying in a hospital bed looking... awful! Mind you it shows that a positive attitude can truly get you through anything.

Acknowledgements

Thank you, thank you, thank you to Alan and Molly. Your unwavering love, support and encouragement fills me with strength and courage, and makes everything possible.

Thanks also to:

Maggie, for constant companionship and canine wisdom.

My family and all my wonderful friends – you know who you are! I am so blessed to have you in my life.

The Beatson West of Scotland Cancer Care Centre, the Western Infirmary, Gartnavel Hospital, The Royal Infirmary, Stobhill hospital, and The Queen Elizabeth University Hospital, Glasgow. I am so grateful to all the medical staff that looked after me, both in hospital and at home.

All the lovely people at Maggie's Centre, for all their advice and assistance.

All the fundraisers, volunteers, and research teams that work tirelessly in this field.

The NHS, for all the fabulous services and voucher schemes it provides.

Duncan Lockerbie at Lumphanan Press for just being brilliant!

And finally, most importantly, to you for taking the time to read this. Wishing you much health and happiness always.